Lick it!

Fix Her Appetite Switch

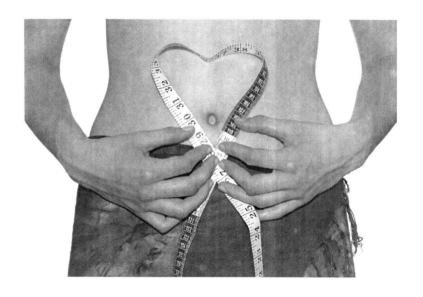

Anne Katherine

Alternate Title

IF the title of this book offends you, you can rip off the cover and this page to expose the following alternative title page.

Her Appetite Switch

Help Her Fix It (and Be a Hero)

Anne Katherine, MA

Best-selling author of *Boundaries, Anatomy of a Food Addiction, When Misery is Company,* and *How to Make Almost Any Diet Work*

First published by Dog Ear Publishing
4010 W. 86th Street, Ste H
Indianapolis, IN 46268
www.dogearpublishing.net

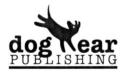

ISBN: 978-159858-713-5

This book is printed on acid-free paper.

Printed in the United States of America

Books by Anne Katherine

Boundaries, Where You End and I Begin

Anatomy of a Food Addiction

Where to Draw the Line

When Misery is Company

How to Make Almost Any Diet Work

Your Appetite Switch (To be available soon)

Penumbra, a Soul's Journey (To be available soon)

www.master**your**appetite.com

www.annekatherine.org

Endorsements

"*Lick It!* is the funniest, most helpful book on food addiction I've yet seen. It should be must reading for anyone who is living with or is friends with a food addict (which is probably the majority of the population!)."

…Christiane Northrup, MD

Dr. Christiane Northrup is the author of *Mother-Daughter Wisdom* (Bantam, 2005), *The Wisdom of Menopause* (Bantam, revised 2006), and *Women's Bodies, Women's Wisdom* (Bantam, revised 2006).

"Light-hearted, fun, scientific—does this really describe a book on appetite disorder? It does when Anne Katherine is the author. This is the most fun you'll ever have learning the brain chemistry that causes people to overeat, and how to help them. If you've ever wondered what to do when someone you love keeps gaining weight, this is the answer. You can really make a difference and be a hero."

…Scott Edelstein

Scott Edelstein, longtime writer, editor, writing teacher, and consultant, knows books. He's published 15 books and over 150 short pieces, on subjects that include psychology, health, writing, art, education, and spirituality. His most recent book is *The Complete Writer's Kit* (Running Press, 2005). He's currently writing two books: one on mental illness and recovery from addiction, to be published by Hazelden, and *Sex and the Spiritual Teacher*, to be published by Wisdom Publications.

"In the last decade, we've learned that family members have the power to support—or sabotage—another family member trying to overcome a behavioral disorder. Anne Katherine's badly needed and easy-to-read new book, *Lick It, Fix Her Appetite Switch*, shows readers what works and what doesn't in helping someone else lose weight. Learn about appetite disorder and understand what can help her eat differently. Buy this book if you're sick of riding the binge-dieting roller coaster along with your loved one."

…Randi Kreger

Randi Kreger is the author of *Stop Walking on Eggshells* (with co-author Paul Mason), *The ABC's of BPD* (with co-author Erik Gunn), and *Love and Loathing* (with co-author Kim A. Williams).

How many times have we seen family and friends sabotage the efforts of a loved person who is struggling to control her weight? How often may we have unintentionally done this ourselves? How much do we wish we knew how to be more supportive? Here is the book that tells us how!"

…Dr. Susan E. Johnson

Dr. Johnson is the author of *When Women Played Hardball* and *Staying Power.*

Gratitude and Dedication

Have I actually ever done the hard things entirely on my own?

I auditioned (trembling) for the Philharmonic Orchestra, yes. But only because my friend Dusty said, "Go ahead, do it, and then when I'm home I can hear you play."

I made it to graduate school, yes. But only because Dean extolled the virtues of Peabody College, Pat pushed me to take the Graduate Record Exam, and Flo came to my apartment, stood over me until I filled in all the blanks, typed the application for me, and took it to the post office.

I hung out my first shingle as a therapist, leaving the security of regular paid employment, but only because Marge taught me how to really make a difference to my clients, Cathy was a vociferous cheerleader, and they let me share their inexpensive office space.

I fell into recovery and got a clear mind, yes, but only due to a compassionate intervention by May C, and the support of Shirley, Dottie Dow, and many recovery friends.

I started writing from an niggling inner voice, yes, but I became a serious writer when May C insisted that my writing was golden and Alliene offered me a cozy apartment in the basement of her home in the Appalacian mountains. She and Betty fostered the most tranquil years of my life in that beautiful world and brought me into their gritty and profoundly holy mountain community. Cradled in safety, I could spin words into cloth.

I continue to write because that inner voice keeps nagging me, yes, but Scott Edelstein, secret service protective detail disguised as literary agent keeps asserting that I'm on another cutting edge, and Sherry keeps washing the dishes, vacuuming the cat hair, and making me laugh. Sherry and Pat Matthews believe so deeply in my work that I can't disbelieve in myself. Jill and Kevin are nestled in my heart and, with Sherry A, Pat, Sherry B, Barbara, Fran, and the AB's are my living family.

And I get to focus on words because other people prop up the infrastructure. Rabbitt keeps fixing my computer, and St. Stephen's Episcopal Church keeps praying for me. Barbara feeds the cats when I'm off learning, Harry is an expert on all things mechanical, Joan Haigh is as good as a library, and Blaine Haigh provides transportation and comic relief. Susan Johnson and Connie Wolfe have great ideas for third drafts, Katie pushes me into musical pursuits, Zim sharpens my bridge game and therefore my mind, as do Jean, Marilyn, Ron, Pat and Doc, John, John, and Kay. Milli and Christine create sugar-free treats, Lynette and Rob keep our office as warm as a kitchen parlor, and my clients stimulate my heart, mind and my creativity. Yvonne, Susan, and the AIG offer me ways out of my aig-shell. Lynn and Rick light up my heart, my antique buddies—Abe, Cassie, Dusty, and Jabber—are my bedrock and touchstones, and Bella is the child of my heart.

In fact, I can look back over my life and see how each bridged precipice was preceeded by the kind and, sometimes, vigorous support of good people, often with no returning profit intended or expected. From my first week of life to the previous 15 minutes, my path has been sustained by the living stones beneath my feet.

It's fitting, therefore, that I dedicate this book to you, the reader. For you, like Alliene, Alice, Betty, and my grandmother, are willing to extend yourself for the sake of someone you care about. You are willing to learn about a condition that has played havoc with the quality of her or his life and to find out what you can do to help.

Without the support of people like you, who among us would have accomplished anything at all? Thank you for joining the elite legion of kind and gracious people.

Reader, I dedicate this book to you.

Table of Contents

1

The Burgled Brownie

Heading home after a long day, you're looking forward to stretching out in your favorite chair, flicking the remote, and munching a couple of leftover brownies—your evening is planned.

But you get home and there are no brownies. There are no cookies. No chips. No dip. It's all gone. It's as if an ant colony has swarmed through your kitchen and nibbled it bare.

Two possibilities: she's on another diet. She's not on a diet.

If she's on another diet, you're in for a week of cabbage soup, no desserts, and strange Styrofoam crackers. If she's not on a diet, the shelf life of sweets and snacks is a millisecond.

What's a husband to do—or a mother, a sister, a best friend, a lover, or a partner? What do you do when you love someone who overeats?

You can rant, you can manipulate her, you can try to control her, or you can get smart.

Ranting is fun. You deserve to have a little tantrum about the frustrations of loving or living with an overeater. It *is* annoying to cope with all the ups and downs of each new diet. Your routine gets interrupted. The comfortable meals you usually eat are pulled from the menu, and the kitchen acquires alien foods.

Manipulation gives you something to do. You can shower her with recipes. You can try controlling her intake by the foods you buy or cook or by fixing her plate for her.

Perhaps you've tempted her with happy endings such as a promised cruise or shopping spree. Or ignited her competitive impulses with talk about how good her high school rival looks now that *she's* dropped 200 pounds.

How about scary stories? You did tell her, didn't you, about the neighbor lady who let herself go and now her husband has run off with his anorectic secretary, Brad.

Probably the most commonly-used tool for influencing an overeater is shame. "You'd look so good if you lost all that weight. You used be so pretty. Do you think you should be wearing yellow? You don't need that biscuit. Wearing shorts—at your weight? You look just like Aunt Heftie—she was a blimp too, but she had the good sense to stay home and not make people look at her."

Strangely enough, shame doesn't work. If it did, every overweight person would be size medium before the end of the year, because I guarantee you, there's not an overweight American who hasn't been shamed enough to turn his toes purple.

This is an experiment that has been exhaustively tested. *Shaming does not work*. Instead, it backfires, sending the person into secret eating as soon as possible, because eating gives them comfort. (Eating for comfort, that's only a part of the problem but it is a significant part and we'll talk about that later.)

Here's the reality: if you want to have impact on the overeater in your life, get smart. Learn about the disorder and understand what can help her to eat differently.

Think also about what you would like for yourself. Check the ones that fit:

❒ When you eat together, would you like consistency around what she can eat and what you can share with her?

❒ Would you like to have consistent limits and freedoms around what you can expect from the kitchen?

❒ Would you like to know what would truly help?

❒ Would you like to be eating healthier yourself?

❒ Do you find yourself being pulled away from your own sensible food plan when her eating gets wild?

❒ Do you want relief from worrying about her health?

❒ Do you want to be able to share more experiences with her?

❐ Are there activities or jaunts you would like to share with her that get curtailed or cancelled because of her eating, weight, or body image?

In this book, you'll get factual, scientific information about the disease of overeating and how you can be of tremendous help. And I'll tell you point blank what doesn't help. I'll also give you tips about each of the above issues so that you can be getting more of what *you* want.

(By the way, I'm going to consistently use female pronouns when referring to the overeater. We all know that both genders overeat, but more women than men do so, and it's just easier to pick the statistical majority than to make awkward *she/he* or *s/he* constructions.)

[Americans can invent anything except an all-gender pronoun.]

2
Get Smart

Overeating has lots of labels such as bulimia, compulsive overeating, binge eating, and binge eating disorder. The problem with each of these is that they put the spotlight on the *behavior* of eating. This misdirection has influenced everyone to target the observable behavior, instead of what *causes* the overeating.

You know what the most commonly applied remedy is—a diet. Diets have been the preferred method of treatment for more than a hundred years and they still don't work. It's not that the diets are bad, it's that they are applied at the wrong end of the problem.

It'd be like trying to cure colds by changing the brand of tissue, as if the runny nose were the heart of the problem instead of the virus causing the overflowing sinuses.

A person eats too much. A diet tries to get that person to eat less. But the real question is, why does she *want* to eat too much? What is driving the eating?

Here is the answer.

Four primary forces drive eating:
1. Hunger
2. Appetite biochemicals
3. Need for comfort
4. Addictive brain chemicals

Any one of these forces can make a person eat. When a woman needs comfort from food, she will eat—whether or not she's hungry. A woman addicted to chocolate will grab some fudge even if she's happy and her appetite is satisfied.

Paste these forces together so that any two or three of them are driving her, and she *will* eat—no matter what you do.

This is why the urge to overeat outlasts even the best-designed diet. The drive to eat is powerful. It is difficult to interrupt unless it is done in a scientific way.

3

Hunger

Empty tummy, low blood sugar, we all know what hunger feels like. Right?

Maybe not. Some overeaters haven't been hungry for years. Their eating has prevented hunger. Thus, hunger is not a large factor in causing most overeaters to binge.

They may have a *fear* of hunger, disguising a fear of emptiness that overeating protects them from. Lots of us, not just overeaters, fear the experience of emptiness—like an internal hollowness—and use all sorts of things to protect ourselves from the risk of it. Sports, television, drinking, attempts at manipulation or control, overworking, meanness, looking outward instead of inward, busyness, computer gaming, gambling—our world offers endless options for distraction.

An overeater uses food. Eating can be an effective distraction from the experience of hollowness or emptiness or any other feeling we don't want to face.

Meanwhile, the most important thing about hunger in her case is for her to be able to tell the difference between hunger and appetite. The remedy for excessive, inappropriate hunger is different in most cases from the remedies for excessive appetite.

If she's participating in my *Master Your Appetite* program (www.master**your**appetite.com) or reading the companion book to this one, *Your Appetite Switch*, then she's already working on this.

If she isn't working on some sort of recovery program, ask her if she's willing to read this book along with you to see if she likes the principles enough to get the companion book. The two of you can follow the suggestions together.

How You Can Help

Begin to explore the difference between hunger and appetite for yourself.

Hunger is experienced as an empty stomach or a hollow feeling in your lower chest. Low blood sugar is another aspect of hunger. Symptoms include headache, feeling light-headed, loss of energy, fuzzy thinking, slower decision-making, crankiness, and difficulty with mental tasks that are usually easy for you.

Appetite isn't located in the stomach, but starts as complex brain activity that leads to unconscious behaviors that are all focused on getting and eating food. It can show up in a variety of ways.

Appetite Signals:

- Interest in food or eating eclipsing other aspects of an occasion such as the people or activities
- Intrusive food thoughts
- Mental pictures of a food or restaurant
- Appearing to function while actually preoccupied with plans to eat
- Wanting a certain food very much
- Feeling driven to eat
- Eating without being able to stop
- Being very conscious of the serving sizes that other people are getting, particularly if their serving of pie, garlic bread, pasta, or nachos is bigger than your own
- Being distracted from the conversation at the table by someone else's unfinished dessert or garlic bread
- Devouring a bag of chips without realizing it until the bag is empty
- Continuing to eat after feeling full
- Browsing kitchen cabinets or the fridge almost as if you were sleepwalking

Other Differences

When you're hungry, almost any food will do, but "solid" food is usually preferred—meat, protein, salad, nuts, raw vegetables. Appetite usually wants a *particular* food—not just the week-old bread but fresh, hot garlic bread, not just any ice cream but moose trails ice cream from the Dairy Princess on Front Street.

If you're really hungry, you'll take the food in front of you. Appetite convinces you to drive out of your way to the Dairy Princess even if it will make you a little late for your rendezvous with your friend—or it'll make you call her to see if she'd be willing to have dinner there, instead of at the health food restaurant she originally suggested.

Hunger is on a rheostat. It's like a dimmer switch that moves from slightly peaked to starving. Appetite is more like a toggle switch. It's either on or off. (Exception: food addiction adds extra settings—craving and gimme-more. A food craving can range from slight to irresistibly intense.)

Do:

- Talk with her about what you're learning for yourself regarding the difference between hunger and appetite.
- Listen to her talk about what she's learning for herself.
- Appreciate her efforts to make these discriminations for herself.

Don't:

- Don't tell her when she's hungry or when her appetite is kicking in.
- Don't make her discriminations for her.

4
Appetite

Most people who overeat do so because their appetite chemicals are out of whack. They are driven to eat by these chemicals, some of which are so powerful that mind-over-matter isn't feasible. Hence, some common advice offered by non-overeaters is about as effective as a Pamper on an elephant—it's just not big enough to cover the job.

Useless Advice

1. Just push yourself away from the table. *(Overeaters don't usually overeat at the table. They eat in their cars, on their couches, at their desks, in their LaZboys.)*
2. Just eat half of what is on your plate. *(If it's on the plate, it's hers. Possession is nine tenths of the law.)*
3. Just take one bite of the pie and leave the rest. *(Not going to happen.)*
4. Brush your teeth as soon as you've finished dinner, then you won't want anymore. *(Like a little toothbrush is going to stop things.)*
5. Don't eat food that starts with a "c" unless it's green. *(Funny.)*
6. Only eat when you're hungry. *(She may not have been hungry for a very long time.)*
7. You don't have to eat anything. Just sit and keep me company while I eat. *(The visual stimulus will start her appetite chemicals aflowing and if your food is ambrosial, forget it.)*

8.   Turn three times counterclockwise, rub your tummy in a spiral, and sit facing the equator before eating. *(Just about as effective as any of the other ideas on this list.)*

* * *

I love to snorkel. Occasionally I see a fish I want to get closer to. If only I could hold my breath, dive deeper, and stay under long enough to follow that fish around awhile, say twenty minutes. I'm not asking for a lot. I just want to hold my breath for 20 minutes and then, I promise, I'll come back to the surface and breathe.

Doesn't work that way. I can try to hold my breath, even if I have a good reason for it—such as being stuck in traffic behind a diesel smoker—and my own body will force me to breathe.

Appetite chemicals work the same way. They are strong and powerful. If appetite chemicals are forcing a person to eat, she will eat. She can't talk herself out of it. You can't talk her out of it. And no bribe or punishment will outlast their influence.

Let's take **NPY** as an example. **Neuropeptide Y** causes a person to eat more food for a longer period than she intends to.

Neuropeptide Y is a chain of 36 amino acids. It is the most potent of appetite stimulators.[i] When it is released in the feeding centers of the brain, it makes a person eat. It also tells the body to stop burning calories. When NPY is repeatedly released, it rapidly induces obesity.[ii]

> **Definitions**
>
> **Peptide**
> A chain of amino acids.
> **Amino Acids**
> The primary components of protein.
> **Protein**
> What a steak is mostly made of. Proteins are composed of amino acids and peptides.

If NPY is pushing your woman's appetite, there is nothing you can do to stop her from eating. It'd be like trying to hold your breath for twenty minutes, or trying to keep yourself from needing a bathroom for three days. You just can't do it. When the contest is between will and body chemicals, body chemicals always win in the long run.

Think Seattle Mariners against the Little League. Oops, bad example. (I'm kidding Seattle; you know I love ya.) Think New York Yankees against your local Little League team.

You can now understand one of the reasons that most diets aren't enduring. Will power can't outlast the pressure exerted by body chemicals.

There are eight ways[iii] the brain can miscue a person to eat too much. If even one of these is operating, she will overeat and probably gain weight. If more than one are influencing her, then she is being driven by a gang of chemicals. They are the engine, she is the passenger, and you are the caboose.

What's the way out of this?

The Exit

- Understand each of the appetite chemicals and how they work.
- Influence the chemicals themselves, doing the things that decrease appetite chemicals and increase satiety (stop-eating) chemicals.
- Support her in these smart interventions.
- Avoid actions on your part that increase *her* appetite chemicals.
- Encourage a program of appetite intervention that makes *one change at a time* in an intelligent order.

5

Appetite Stoppers

The body has a counter-measure to appetite, and this is satiety. Satiety chemicals tell a person to stop eating.

Just as appetite operates differently than hunger, satiety is different from fullness. Satiety stops appetite, while fullness stops hunger.

Fullness, like hunger, can be experienced from within. They are both sensations. Satiety, like appetite, can't be felt as a sensation. It is a drive (or the absence of one) that shows up in a person's behavior.

Normal people have an increase in appetite as a mealtime approaches, and then as they begin eating, satiety chemicals kick in and tell them when they've eaten enough.

If this is not happening, something in the person's history, genes, or daily practices is interfering. The women I coach are mystified when I describe satiety. They can't find a time when they haven't had an interest in eating. Only when they've been on their program for about a month, do they start to realize what satiety is like. That's a very happy day for them.

If satiety chemicals are not working, a woman has no natural internal message that causes her to lose interest in food and turn to something else. Thus, she can continue to eat for hours.

A person who overeats has a defect in satiety. There are three satiety chemicals that we can influence so that a person's internal appetite stopper is restored: peptide YY, serotonin, and cholecystokinin.

Do:

Imagine what it would be liked to be pushed to do something and to have no internal message to stop. Imagine—pushed to do something, pushed, pushed, and to have to make yourself stop against all that pressure. It'd be like placing your hands flat on the nose of a loaded semi and trying to push it backwards up a hill.

Here's the value of finding something in your own life that is a similar experience. When she starts following a program to balance her appetite chemicals, she'll be doing something very, very hard. She'll be changing a bodily state that has been in charge of her for many years.

It's difficult.

If you can feel, from the inside, just how hard it is, you might see how important you are to her. You can help her and make a huge difference. At the least, you can refrain from doing things that would make her effort even more difficult.

6

Appetite Chemical 1

NPY—Neuropeptide Y

In a previous chapter, you were introduced to the power of NPY, one of the brawniest appetite drivers. The question now is, what causes these little tyrants to flood the feeding centers?

The answer—fasting. Repeated bouts of calorie restriction—through extreme diets, anorexia, or self neglect—make the body wary of being deprived. Over time, it institutes countermeasures more and more quickly. NPY is one of these.

NPY doesn't bother her while she's delaying or skipping meals. It lurks. It waits. It bides its time. When she finally gets around to eating, that's when it strikes, making her want extra food and pushing her to eat all of it.

Clever, really. And the body *is* clever. The body's logic is this: if this tender human creature lives in a world of periodic famine, pump in the nutrition when food does show up.

Thus, a person's body can become so sensitive to fasting that her system reacts to the first sign of food scarcity—even so minor an event as a delayed meal. Plus, a person who is active while fasting—exercising before breakfast, for example—will accumulate even more NPY.

Ironically, women who eat too much are notorious for skipping breakfast and even lunch, for working or shopping too long before eating, and for delaying meals. This sets them up to eat too much—and to gain weight.

What this means for her:

- She should never skip a meal, not ever.
- She should always eat breakfast.
- If a meal is to be delayed, she should eat a small protein snack.

Do:

- Encourage her to eat breakfast.
- Encourage her to eat lunch.
- Encourage her to eat dinner.
- If a meal is to be delayed, bring her a small protein snack and encourage her to eat it.
- Have protein snacks on hand, such as individually wrapped cheeses, unsalted almonds, or soy milk. You know what she likes (or is allergic to).
- Prepare for situations that could delay a meal:
  - If you're traveling, look for a restaurant well ahead of the usual meal time, or pack snacks that travel well or are allowed on planes.
  - If you know that Aunt Tippler always serves dinner late cause she gets tanked in the kitchen, have a mini-meal before you go.
  - Keep a little supply of snacks in the car in case you run into traffic on your way to a dinner or party.
  - Go early so you can eat before the show instead of after.

Don't:

- Never ridicule her for eating. Shaming her for eating will cause her to feel that she's wrong any time she eats, and this will lead to skipping meals and that, as you now know, will set her up to be enslaved by NPY.
- Never eat up all her snacks. Always leave a day's supply for her and replace what you've eaten before the next day.
- Avoid situations that cause delayed meals.
- Don't let anyone else get away with a snide remark about her eating, like the classic, *"Are you eating again?"*

Do:

- Shut down any shaming like the hero you are.
- Look at this example of support:

"Grandpa, stop it. It's not okay to talk to my wife (daughter, sister, friend) that way. She's on a special program. Leave her alone."

Grandpa: *"Oh, I didn't know she/you were so sensitive."*

You: *"Most people are when they are put down. So stop it."*

7

Satiety (Stop Eating) Chemical 1

PYY–Polypeptide YY

Peptide YY is a 36 amino acid chain that (mostly) inhibits eating. When Peptide YY levels rise, appetite falls and eating stops.[iv]

PYY opposes NPY. NPY is on the offensive team and PYY is on the defense. NPY pushes toward the goal of more food and PYY blocks that forward advance.

When normal people eat, 15 minutes into the meal, their plasma levels of PYY begin to rise and plateau about 75 minutes later. Also their PYY levels peak in proportion to the amount of food they eat.[v] The more they eat, the more PYY enters their system, and it makes them stop eating after they've had an appropriate portion of food.

When our bodies receive regular doses of PYY, our food intake will normally be reduced by 33% over 24 hours.

However, each time a person fasts (goes on an extreme diet), her PYY is suppressed and smaller amounts are released after eating.[vi] Thus, her natural appetite stopper diminishes with each succeeding diet.

Remember those protein fasts that were the rage 20 years ago? (Oh, wait. I saw one advertised last week.) Can you imagine what happened to the NPY and PYY in the bodies of those thousands of patients who fasted for six months?

NPY stockpiled like arms proliferation. And PYY disappeared. Makes more sense out of that 95% failure rate for fasting diets.

If the person you loved fell prey to such a diet, afterwards, she probably re-gained the lost weight and then some. So did thousands of others.

95% failure in sustaining weight loss after a fast, for obvious chemical reasons, and they are still available. Would we accept such odds with a cell phone company? How about if our cars broke down on a certain scheule? Or the refrigerator broke right after the warranty expired. Ooops, bad examples. Darn, maybe we *will* accept a high failure rate.

Research shows that when obese and lean bodies were compared, the large bodies were deficient in PYY, both when not eating and after eating. [vii] People carrying extra weight had a deficiency of this satiety chemical. Their bodies weren't sending them a message to stop eating, because the messenger quit.

Normal people have a peak in PYY levels after breakfast, lunch, and supper, but obese subjects show a delayed peak, long after a large evening meal.[viii] This explains their tendency to skip breakfast. They reach satiety overnight and awaken with their appetites suppressed, which works against them. Skipping breakfast causes a rise in NPY. This forces them to eat too much later in the day, perpetuating the cycle.

A Wary Brain

Just as you can't hold your breath for 20 minutes even when you have a good reason, you can't make yourself be uninterested in food if NPY is pushing you and PYY is inactive.

The body is pointed non-stop toward survival. It never takes a break. It also has ways of remembering repeated threats to survival. It catches on rapidly if a certain threatening condition repeats itself, and then it creates systems to deal with that threat.

Remember, food being available in mountainous heaps is only a recent condition and only in certain countries at that. Prior to modern times, food scarcity was the norm for a thousand centuries. Thus the body perceives fasting as a threat. What we call a diet, the body calls starvation, and it has many automatic defenses against starvation and very few against too much food.

Extra weight is actually a magnificent project that our species developed to ensure personal survival. Even a world-famous diet will not be enough, by itself, to overcome the ramparts erected by the body. In the long term, the body must be convinced that its survival is not being threatened.

The body is hard-wired to promote species survival as well, and the species is more concerned about female starvation than male. The male body is used to hunting large territories on small amounts of dried food. Even if a man is malnourished, he can still breed, but, from nature's viewpoint, women must always be protected in case they get pregnant.

In the early 1980s, when we began wondering what had caused the cascade of eating disorders among American women, we found one initiating event that most disordered eaters shared: an extreme diet. During their teen years, mostly, women had restricted their food intake.

From the body's point of view, this was the worst possible timing. Just when a female was approaching her prime baby-making years, she was starving.

Alarm! Call out the troops! Stockpile NPY. Lower metabolism. Stop fabricating PYY.

The body's 911 response created an increase in fat storage and appetite, and a decrease in energy and satiety. (The reluctance to move often found in large people is related to this policy of sparing energy.)

So what happened? Women ate more and became heavier. This spurred them to try new diets. Each time they did, they further scared their bodies, especially if a diet was extreme. Before very long, their bodies were permanently armed against starvation.

Fast forward twenty years and you find these women with extra weight, a chemically caused resistance to exercise, and bodies defended against calorie burning.

What This Means for Her

- She must have 2 small snacks a day, mid-morning and mid-afternoon.
- Snacks must include protein and should not include anything made with sugar, flour, wheat, or any artificial sweetener except for stevia.

In her book, (*Your Appetite Switch*) or program (www.master-yourappetite.com), she has a list of legal snacks and a stepped progression of snack ingredients that supports her self-diagnostic process. Before she settles into her permanent snack guidelines, you'll have to check with her to see what snacks are allowed this week.

Do:

- Support her snacking program.
- Encourage her to get her snack when snack time rolls around.
- Offer to bring her her snack.
- Offer to prepare legal snacks.
- Help replenish snacks.
  - ○ You can find a variety of prepared snack vegetables at the food market. Rinse these before distributing them to smaller snack bags or containers. (Prepared vegetables can have a high bacterial count the longer they sit on a market shelf, even if the handling conditions were excellent.)
  - ○ Celery and carrots will stay fresher if you add water to the storage container (but they have to be eaten within the week).
  - ○ A variety of cheeses come already sliced and individually packaged in snack sizes.
  - ○ Be sure you get yogurt that isn't sweetened by sugar, corn syrup, or aspartame (NutraSweet, or Equal).
  - ○ Distribute a large bag of unsalted almonds into little snack bags.
  - ○ Grill or bake more meat than needed for a family meal, slice it, and divide it into snack bags.

8

Ashamed to Eat

One of the biggest problems I've had in counseling overeaters is getting them to eat snacks. When I developed my first programs for overeaters in the 1970's, I naively believed they'd love it when I gave them permission to eat. I thought by saying, "Eat your snacks," they'd dive in. In one of my programs, clients could even earn a free massage if they racked up enough 'positive action' points each month. The catch? They could make the required point count only by eating their snacks.

I never paid for a single massage. That was one of my early lessons that body chemistry will overtrump a good idea every time.

Here's the reality:
- She must snack (following the criteria in the previous chapter) in order to rebuild her PYY.
- She can very easily be distracted from maintaining her snacking program.

Here are the dangers:
- Someone will shame her for snacking.
  If someone makes a cruel, ignorant remark about how often she's eating, she'll drop it like a hot potato.
- She will run out of her snack foods.
  Obviously, as she consumes her snacks, they will run out. If, between work, childcare, parent care, household tasks, and commuting, she is too busy to think about her own needs, she may forget to buy more snack materials and may put off organizing snacks for easy use.

- Snacking interferes with a food addiction.
  *Food addiction is another powerful cause of disordered appetite.
  If she is addicted to certain foods, she'll be resistant to fostering
  chemicals that remove her desire to eat.*
- Snacking interferes with her structure for daily comfort.
  *She may have a pattern of saving eating till later so that she
  can dive into food as into a safety net or warm cave of comfort.*
- She will resist snacking out of an entrenched belief that
  she's not supposed to eat.

Overeaters tend to have a deep-seated perspective that all
eating is bad and that not-eating is good. Never mind that this is
what got her into this problem to begin with (restricting foods, dieting). It's hard for any of us to change our mindsets, especially if
we're caught in a cycle of self blame and poor self esteem.

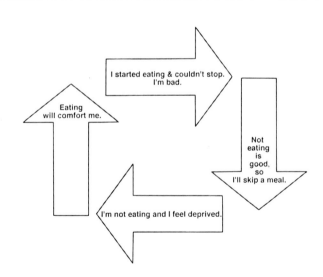

The Cycle of Self Blame

Do:

- Remember that by snacking, she is restoring her satiety. If she gets into the self-blame cycle, help her step out by reminding her of the reality of her body chemistry.
- Protect her. If someone ridicules her for eating, stand up for her.
- Get in the habit of picking up legal snacks for her when you're in a store.

Don't:

- Never tease her, not even in the slightest way, about eating.
  I promise you, this is a very, very tender trigger. It may seem hilarious to you; it will be catastrophic for her.
- Don't eat up her snacks. Replace, on that same day, any that you consume.

9

You Don't Have to Be a Chemist

Curious?
Why do people eat when they're already full?
If she smells pastry, can she think clearly about not eating it?
How are smell neurons different from other sensory neurons?

You don't have to be a biology teacher or a doctor to understand that chemicals are powerful. Motor oil, bleach, tobacco, coffee, fertilizer, cough syrup, Coca Cola—these are all chemicals. You pick the one that has the properties you need, and count on it to do a job.

Your body is full of chemicals. They each have a job, and they work together (and sometimes they oppose each other) to keep your body running.

Definitions

Food triggers—Foods that stimulate appetite.
Sight triggers—Pictures of food or food displays that stimulate appetite.
Smell triggers—Food aromas that stimulate appetite.

You may think that you want to eat just because you're hungry. But you can want to eat even if you're not hungry. After a balanced breakfast of juice, an omelet, and toast, you can still walk past a tray of jelly donuts and grab one.

It's not from hunger, because you were full.

It's from appetite.

How could you have an appetite so soon after breakfast? From the sight of tempting food.

Just the sight or smell of food can release appetite chemicals in your brain.[ix] So that, without even thinking about it, you can reach out and grab a donut, even though you're full.

Without even thinking about it, a person can eat something if her appetite has been stimulated.

Do

- Help her avoid the sight and smell of tempting food.
- Before any situation with lots of tempting food (fairs, parties, banquets, holiday events, the mall food court), ask if she'd like your help avoiding sight and smell triggers. If she says yes, you can help in these ways:
  - ○ Scout out the food selections for her, and note where her dangerous foods are. (In Chapter 19, I'll explain what kinds of foods might be dangerous for her.)
  - ○ Tell her where her safety zones are. (These will be places in the room, or sections of the buffet table, that have foods she can eat.)
  - ○ Offer to fix her plate for her so that she doesn't even have to expose herself to her trigger foods.
  - ○ Eat at a distance from the food vendors. At the mall, take your trays out of the food court and sit by the fountain. At a fair, walk away from the food booths. At a party, opt for the chairs that face away from the buffet. Find the furthest table from the dessert bar, and sit facing the other direction.
  - ○ If the cash register is on top of a display case containing pastries, cookies, or candies, you pay the bill while she waits by the door.

10

Triggered Appetite

You can skip this chapter if you want. It's more info about the brain mechanics behind appetite stimulation. *But if you still think it's her fault that she eats too much, consider this section required reading.*

Food smells are potent appetite stimulators. You probably know that some restaurants funnel appetizing smells into the street to draw people in. You can enter a restaurant without realizing that you have been seduced.

Why does this work?

Because the nerves that carry aromas into the brain bypass your thinking centers. They go straight to the animal brain so that you react without conscious awareness.

This was handy when your ancestors lived in caves. If they smelled a bear, they grabbed a spear without hesitation. They didn't have to puzzle out the name of the creature or what they should do. They reacted milliseconds faster, and this saved their lives so they could raise your great great great x 500 greats great grandfather.

Even today, this feature alerts you. The smell of smoke, natural gas, or gasoline in the wrong situation puts you on instant guard.

Unfortunately for your loved one, this attribute causes her trouble. Aromas of popcorn at the movies, fried food, and baking can all create instant cravings that are difficult to resist. Such smells make you *want* that food—that frying bacon, that fresh-baked bread, that chocolate.

We can't think our way out of this. Since the smell neurons (nerves) bypass our brain's thinking centers, we will go toward that aromatic food and forget any previous plans or promises.

The way to prevent this is to move out of range of such smells immediately. If you know you're headed toward that spot on Main Street where the candy store vents its kitchen, cross the street or go around the block.

The sight of food is marginally less evocative. Here we have some choice if we remove the stimulus immediately. Sight sensors do traverse the thinking part of the brain, which gives us time to close our eyes and turn away.

However, the longer we expose ourselves to the sight of tempting food, the more powerful it becomes. Plus, its triggering power increases if we see other people eating and enjoying it.

A cake sitting on a counter isn't as powerful a trigger as a group of people laughing while they share a similar cake. (At least, it's not so powerful as long as you don't smell the cake and you turn away quickly.)

A food that is a symbol of celebration and well-being will almost always have more triggering power. (Contrast a hot dog in a pan of water on your stove with a ballpark hotdog, fans cheering and the crack of a bat in the background.)

She may avoid ice cream easily when she's home, yet be desperate for it when you're vacationing at that little seaside resort with the homemade ice cream parlor. If she walks by while they're baking waffle cones or looks at all the fancy ice creams in the display case, her appetite chemicals are certain to be triggered.

Movies, commercials, TV programs, food ads, and pictures on menus can all trigger appetite.

Being Her Super Hero

If you're willing to go the extra mile, here are some other ways you can expand her safety zone. (But ask her first, and only do the things that she wants you to.)

- Go through her magazines and rip out the food ads, food pictures (except for salad, fish, and similar non-triggering food), and recipes.

- When a food commercial comes on TV, flip to another channel.
- If a movie shows people eating tempting food, tell her she can close her eyes and you'll let her know when they're done.
- When your restaurant menu has pictures, ask if she'd like you to tell her what the selections are. Or if you are familiar with the restaurant, ask if she'd like to choose her meal before entering the restaurant. (Notice that you're giving her a choice rather than simply taking over.)

She will be enormously grateful for your help, and you will be her hero.

The next two chapters are more about the science of appetite. Feel free to skip them and go straight to Chapter 13. Just looking at the pictures while you turn pages will tell you a lot.

11
Brain Parts

If you're totally sick of science, skip to the next chapter.

Brain Chemistry 101
Neuron
A single nerve cell with fibers that receive (dendrites), a fiber that sends (axon), and a nucleus.

Dendrites
Nerve fibers that *receive* messages. A neuron can have multiple dendrites, and these can branch. A **receptor** is at the very end of a dendrite.

Axon
A nerve fiber that *sends* messages. A neuron has one axon, and this can branch too.

Synapse
The place where an axon meets a dendrite.

Neurotransmitter
The chemical that flows from an axon to a dendrite to deliver a message.

Receptor
The part of a dendrite that *receives* the neurotransmitter.

Neurotransmission
Neuron A gets chummy with neuron B

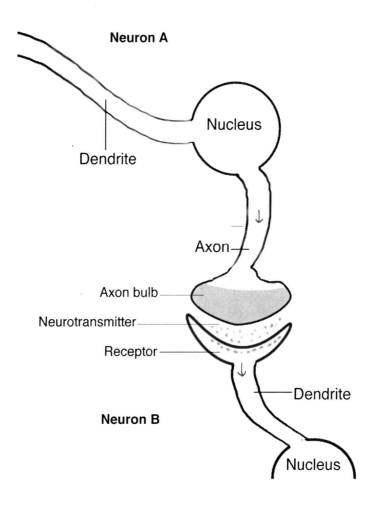

A receptor filling with neurotransmitter and passing on the message.

Receptors and Wrenches

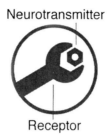

Neurotransmitter

Receptor

A wrench is like a receptor.

A receptor is like a wrench, specially shaped in a chemical sense to receive a specific plug-in that only works if the two match. Just as a wrench has heads designed to fit bolts of precise sizes, each receptor has a particular chemical configuration that responds only to a chemical that is a precise fit. Receptors for Neuropeptide Y, for example, will not respond to milk.

12
Force-feeding

This is an optional chapter. Feel free to skip it if you're fed up with biology. Just notice the pictures—the hypothalamus and loading dock—as you turn the pages.

ENS

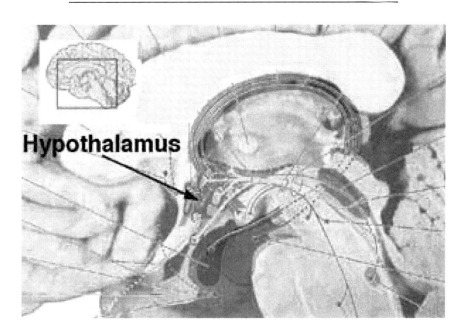

Brain Chemistry 201: The Hypothalamus[x]

You may know that we humans have a central nervous system (CNS) that includes the brain and spinal cord, and a peripheral nervous system (PNS) that operates nearly all the stuff below the neck. But did you also know we each have something called an enteric nervous system? This is the nervous system devoted to nutrition, eating, and elimination of waste.

Compared to the peripheral nervous system, which has a paltry 20,000 nerves heading to the brain, the ENS contains about 100 million neurons. (The body surely likes to guarantee it's gonna get fed.) These nerves connect all the body parts involved in feeding.

The hypothalamus is on the underside of the brain and is a big player in feeding, with at least three areas, and possibly a fourth, that promote eating.

One of these, the paraventricular nucleus is the binge eating center, the "locate an all-you-can-eat, open-24-hours-a-day buffet" button. NPY is one of the chemicals that will trigger it.

In fact, each of the hypothalamic eating centers have numerous **receptors** for NPY which, when stimulated, not only increase eating, but lower a thyroid stimulating hormone, thereby lowering metabolism and energy. The low thyroid levels that many overeaters experience could well be traced to this over-functioning of NPY.

Did I mention she should never skip a meal?

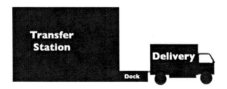

A receptor is like the loading dock at a transfer station.
It receives a delivery and then passes it into the eating center.

13

Stop-Eating Chemical Number 2 & Three Heavies

More Science

Feel free to read just this page and then skip to the Bottom Line.

Satiety chemicals have their own receiving docks in the hypothalamus and some of these are for leptin, a 167-chain amino acid. Fat cells use leptin to tell the body how much fat is stored.

Leptin is like an inventory officer. It goes to one of the hypothalamic eating centers and says, "We have enough fat in storage. Stop eating already!"

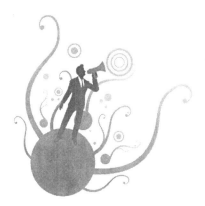

Leptin shouts, "Stop Eating!"

So what's with the leptin in a large person? Studies show that obese folks are either deficient in leptin or have receptors resistant to it.[xi]

It's possible that ghrelin suppresses leptin. Ghrelin is a 28-amino acid peptide released primarily from the stomach in response to fasting. It stimulates eating by acting on the hypothalamus.

Typically, ghrelin peaks with the approach of a meal and falls within an hour after a meal. When it was administered to human subjects, their intake at a buffet increased 30%.[xii] And although eating will cause a decrease in ghrelin levels, one study with rats showed that if a meal is high in fat, the ghrelin level rebounds after the meal.[xiii]

As ghrelin rises, leptin falls. So an eating stimulator waxes at the same time an eating inhibitor wanes.

What can stop this madness? PYY. PYY backs ghrelin off, decreasing food intake by 40% in a buffet study.[xiv]

Then there are orexins A (OX-A) and B (OX–B), which both stimulate eating in the hypothalamus, though OX-A causes more trouble.

Want to guess what causes an increase in orexins? Yep, fasting.

I should probably mention that overeaters shouldn't skip a meal.

Bottom Line

Five of the most powerful chemicals that balance eating are all disturbed by one action—fasting. That includes, for those bodies made sensitive to famine, skipped and delayed meals and extreme diets.

One action fixes these imbalances—eating in a particular way every two to three hours.

14

Not Talking Musical Notes Here

If you love an overeater, you've been up and down the scale, pun intended. She's been frustrated by the numbers on the scale and you've been frustrated too.

I'm sure not going to talk away your irritation, but I hope you can see who really deserves it. Who do you think deserves to be the target of your irritation?

- Diet fads
- Magazines that push dieting
- Extreme diet programs
- A culture that is so appearance-conscious
- Uninformed health systems that promote extreme diets
- Your precious overeater

Each time she went on a diet, she had these chemical processes working against her:

- Over-stimulated hypothalamic feeding centers
- Overactive Orexins
- Excess NPY
- Malfunctioning leptin receptors
- Insufficient leptin
- PYY deficiency
- Excess ghrelin
- Insufficient dopamine D2 receptors (we'll get to this later)

All these chemicals lined up to foil her and with some diets, they were only made worse. I hope you can see that this chemical barrage would always defeat her and that trying to stop it with self-discipline or will power would be like carrying a six-pack of beer in a wet paper bag. It would burst right on through.

Her way out is to understand these chemicals and work with them intelligently. Your way in is to support her exploration, education, and serenity. Don't worry. I'll give you easy ways to do it.

Do:

- Understand that her process will take some time. She has to do three things:
  - ○ Diagnose the chemicals that are out of whack in her body.
  - ○ Reduce the appetite-causing chemicals.
  - ○ Increase the satiety-promoting chemicals
- Understand that she has to do these things in a particular order. She can't do them all at once or she will scare her body into defending appetite.
- Understand that these chemical shifts could start within three weeks of beginning her program, but she will still be tenderly making significant changes three months later.
- Most important: understand that **she will have to keep her program practices going in order for her chemicals to stay balanced.** (It's not like taking an aspirin for a headache—one pill and the problem is gone.)

Don't:

- Don't ask her if she's lost weight yet.
- Don't suggest that she's eating too much. (Once she trusts her snacking program and sees how this changes her appetite, her meals will automatically become smaller.)
- Don't push her to eat.
- Don't try to get her to join you in eating snacks made of sugar, wheat, flour, or diet drinks.

15

The Taste that Kills

Curious?
What common diet advice sets up weight gain?
Can we be fooled into thinking a food is safe?
Can diet sodas cause people to gain weight?

"Instead of using oil, poach fish or chicken slices in bouillon."

" Switch to diet soda, only one calorie."

"Add flavor without adding fat. Stir fry cabbage, carrots, and shallots in broth or bouillon…"

"Try our easy low-cal frozen dinners."

"Start your meal with soup."

Each of the above statements is paraphrased from various diet plans. People wanting to lose weight try hard to follow such advice.

But what if, by doing so, they are not helping themselves? What if they are actually causing their bodies to *gain* weight?

Excited Neurons

One of the ways we can get fooled by the food industry has to do with our automatic trust of words like "natural," "pure," "organic," or "farm raised." I know I was fooled when NutraSweet and Equal flooded the market, and advertisers said, "It's merely a chemical that is already present in the body."

That's true. So is fat. A marketer could wrap up a big cube of fat, slap a price on it, and call it Satis. Take a look. -->

New Product--Satis!

Happy Foods is running a special this week on Satis, a new food derived from organically-fed, free-range livestock raised on small farms.

Satis is chock-full of a naturally occuring body nutrient that is essential for health. Satis will make your skin soft and your hair shiny. It helps your blood clot and controls inflammation. Best of all, it stores energy for you so that when you need it, you'll have it.

Take vitamins? Satis ensures that vitamins A, D, E, and K get to where they're going.

Babies love it--and it's good for them too! Don't miss this special: 3 cubes for only $5.00.

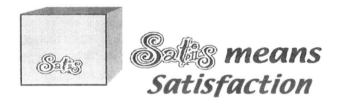

Satis means **Satisfaction**

All claims in this ad are true—except, of course, that there is a product called Satis.

Here's the list of ingredients from a bouillon box sitting on my desk: salt, monosodium glutamate, vegetable oil (palm, sunflower, soybean, cotton seed), sugar, natural flavor, caramel color, onion, spices, disodium guanylate, disodium inosinat, beef meat, turmeric.

If you thought you were getting a nice natural food one step up from beef or chicken stock, think again.

What is glutamate anyway?

[Information in the remaining sections of this chapter is partially derived from the book *Excitotoxins: The Taste that Kills* by Russell l. Blaylock, MD, and is reprinted with permission of Health Press NA Inc., Albuquerque, NM.]

Recipe:
Hydrolyzed Vegetable Protein aka Vegetable Protein, Soy Protein, Natural Flavorings, or Spices

Ingredients
Cart of vegetables unfit for sale
Vat of sulphuric acid
Caustic soda
MSG (optional)

Boil vegetables in acid for one day.
Neutralize acid with caustic soda. (Obtain from soap-maker.) Dry brown sludge to a powder. Add MSG if desired. Add special amino acids for a beefy taste.

Label: Glutamate, aspartate, cysteic acid, Carcinogens, oh my

---

You wouldn't think seaweed has that much call to be excited, but it turns out that the chemical responsible for the flavor-enhancing quality of a Japanese culinary seaweed was glutamate. Chemists discovered that when glutamate was added to food, it suppressed undesirable flavors, hid the tinny taste of canned foods, and made bland food delicious.[xv]

When this news reached the big names in American food production in the middle of the 20th century, they fell on this additive like the Holy Grail and added monosodium glutamate (MSG) to nearly every packaged food they could think of.

Soy protein and vegetable protein sound healthy, don't they. These were among the raft of flavor enhancers that were developed in the wake of MSG. Many of these additive offspring contained up to 40% MSG.[xvi] Take a look at the manufacturing process as described in the box on the left. Do they still seem healthy?

The bubble burst quietly in 1957, when two doctors discovered that glutamate and aspartate imported from outside the body actually destroyed nerves. As further research brought more horror stories, glutamate and aspartate got a new label: neurotoxin.

More Science

Feel free to skip this part if it's too heady. *Skip to the "Diet Soda Fantasy" at the bottom of the page.*

Here's the problem with aspartate and glutamate. The terrible twosome makes nerves get too excited. In an attempt to calm itself, the body uses power vacs to suck out excess excitotoxins. Your power vac plugs into the wall, but the body's vac uses little cellular batteries (Krebs's cycle).

You know how easily batteries burn out. Well, the body's batteries can also burn out. When this happens, the body can't clean up the excess chemicals. Then glutamate and aspartate flood the nerve cells, and the neurons die. It doesn't stop there. Not only does an excess of excitotoxin kill the nerves it touches, it also kills the nerves touched by the flooded neurons.

Do you want to know what wears out the body's batteries? Consuming foods with the additives glutamate or aspartate. The human body is usually capable of handling its own normal amounts of glutamate and aspartate but eating additive amounts taxes the system. (If you want further details, find them on page 39 of Russell Blaylock's book, *Excitotoxins*.)

Eating additives glutamate or aspartate may also increase the risk of Parkinson's, ALS, brain tumors, and migraine headaches—and don't get me started on what it does to pregnant women, babies, and children.

The Diet Soda Fantasy

Your food addict may be quite dependent on diet sodas. She may have been drinking them for years. She may even have been told now and then that diet sodas weren't good for her, yet she kept drinking them.

Diet sodas, for many binge eaters, are a crutch. They are a way to get through the day. They are perceived as a safe treat, because they have few calories. Plus, the caffeine contained in most diet sodas gives an additional boost.

I know from experience that overeaters have great difficulty accepting that diet sodas could be bad for them and even more trouble letting them go. I've written another book for her that gives all the science and research behind the principles in this book called *How to Make Almost any Diet Work*. There, she's been shown the same facts you're getting here. However, my experience is that she will take this data lightly.

Food addicts tend to believe that diet sodas keep them from gaining more weight. The opposite is true. Aspartate can cause the body to hold on to weight. (In fact, if lab rats need to be fattened for obesity studies, they are given msg.)

When NutraSweet and Equal, primarily composed of aspartame (aspartate), flooded the market, dieters welcomed them with open mouths. Yet even though the sodas and desserts made with NutraSweet were sugar-free, they didn't seem to fulfill the promised joy of weight loss. In fact, food addicts who had stayed away from addictive foods and had sustained healthy eating programs for years were suddenly relapsing in droves after drinking these new diet sodas.

Small wonder they didn't lose weight. Excess levels of glutamate have been shown to damage a feeding regulation area of the hypothalamus, causing lots of problems including obesity and decreased fertility.[xvii] Worse, msg passes through the placenta causing obese offspring.

In recent years we've seen an increase in childhood obesity. I wonder if these are children of mothers who innocently drank diet sodas to keep their weight down.

I'm not going to ask you to convince her or to even monitor her soda drinking, but I do want you to have enough information to rebut her if she falls back into the fantasy that diet sodas are good for her. If she defends soda drinking, you'll know the truth and be able to toss her a fact or two to chew on.

Also, it won't help her if you perceive diet sodas as harmless. Remember that they are not.

Bear in mind, obesity caused by hypothalamic lesions is not being caused by eating. This gives a different way to think about the obese child who is taunted by classmates or the adult who has tried diet after diet and felt like a failure—while complying with advice that told her to eat bouillon and frozen diet meals and diet sodas, all of which contained chemicals that made her store weight.

Russell Blaylock wrote, "It is ironic that so many people drink soft drinks sweetened with NutraSweet when aspartate can produce the exact same lesions as glutamate, resulting in gross obesity. (p. 80) [xviii]

The weight caused by aspartate or msg doesn't easily come off. One reason for this may be that these excitotoxins damage receptor cells.

In a previous chapter, you read that leptin helps a person stop eating, and that obese people seem to have a defect in their leptin receptor cells. When such receptor cells are defective, it doesn't matter how much leptin is pumped into the system, the body still won't get the message that it already has enough fat in storage.

This exact result has come from studies with mice. No matter how much leptin they were given, once they had received msg, they could not lose weight and in fact continued to gain. [xix]

Clearly, all of us would do ourselves a favor by avoiding foods containing aspartate and glutamate. But for anyone who tends to overeat, these two products are particularly pernicious.

You may have noticed that foods sweetened by aspartame are quietly disappearing, while Splenda is arriving with little fanfare. Little is known about Splenda, but forgive me for being suspicious about it, since it took 50 years for researchers to figure out the problem with glutamate, and another 40 years for the problem to be brought to public awareness.

However, Stevia, another low-calorie sweetener, is looking good. It appears to actually help balance blood sugar and seems to not trigger excess eating. It's widely available in health food stores. Relatively little is known about Stevia, however, so you would not be unwise to be somewhat cautious.

Don't:

- Never, ever, under any circumstances, offer her a diet drink containing aspartame (Equal or NutraSweet).
- Never buy or offer a NutraSweet food or drink to your person.

Do:

- When you are both eating in a restaurant that has those little blue packets of Equal, you can help by asking the server if they have something less harmful. Even better, carry little green packets of stevia for such situations.
- Eating some protein every two hours and fruit now and then helps a brain to heal. Support her in having regular healthy snacks.
- Magnesium may help heal damage from aspartate and glutamate. Encourage her to take a well-rounded mineral supplement (if her doctor approves).

16

Pausing to Take Stock

You've come a long way. You've now been exposed to a list of chemicals that make her overeat. You've also learned about the antidote: chemicals that make her stop eating.

In a way, it's simple. If the primary cause of her overeating is that her appetite switch is stuck in the on-position, she can remedy this by:

- Strategic snacking
- Never, ever, under any circumstance, missing any meal.
- Never ingesting msg or aspartame.

If she is not addicted to any foods, this is all she needs to do. Within a surprisingly short time, her appetite and satiety chemicals will normalize and, as long as she sustains the above principles, her appetite will calm.

Do support her in perpetuating her program.

However, if she's been driven to eat for more than a decade, it's very likely that additional factors are affecting her. For example, eating for comfort—lots do it, but why does that work?

17

Why Comfort Eating Works

I'm guessing that at some time in your life, something upset you and you swallowed some form of alcohol. You didn't question the mechanism by which alcohol would help you out. It seemed obvious. From experience, perhaps, you knew that alcohol was a substance that altered your feelings.

If somebody said to you, alcohol makes a change in the brain, would you be surprised? I propose that we don't question the machinery of alcohol-induced relief, because alcohol seems like a chemical.

Candy doesn't seem like a chemical. Bread certainly doesn't seem like a chemical. But both are substances that can make changes in the brain, changes separate from that of providing nutrition.

Definitions

Serotonin—
a neurotransmitter that soothes.

Tryptophan—
the amino acid that is the raw ingredient for serotonin.

Certain foods have the capacity to trigger two chemical streams that bring about comfort. The first of these streams operates through serotonin, a neurotransmitter. (Neurotransmitters pass messages between neurons/nerves.)

Eating sugar starts a process that leads to an increase in serotonin.

The outstanding property of serotonin is that it soothes. It promotes relaxation, relief, and sleepiness. So the first consequence of starch and sugar eating is relief of stress through an increase in serotonin.

Naturally, stress and pain relief make an impression. Even little kids have a quick learning curve around the relief that is produced by candy.

Can Eating Make You More Vulnerable to Stress?

Guess what happens as a person turns again and again to sugar or starch for relief? Serotonin gets used up. As serotonin gets depleted, two things happen. Her appetite increases and she becomes more vulnerable to stress.

As she experiences heightened stress, what do you suppose she does? She eats more sugar and starch in an effort to find relief.

Can you see the cycle thus created?

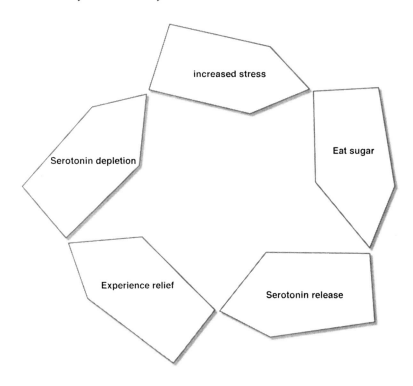

The Stress Cycle

Over time, she becomes ever more vulnerable to stress as her serotonin supply diminishes, simultaneously decreasing satiety as well. Her appetite will automatically increase.

With the body's logic, this makes sense. An important chemical is depleted, so make her eat more.

Eventually, depending on the amount of stress, the degree of support, the composition of a person's neural nets, and her DNA, she may cross a line. More accurately, her brain will develop a new series of connections. When these connections are in place, then the second stream of relief will kick in—addiction.

18
Enter the Addiction

Curious?
Are some people set up to become addicts by virtue of their body chemistry?
Can body chemistry make a person especially responsive to sweet foods?
Can people really become addicted to food?

Addiction is an alteration in brain physiology and anatomy that leads to dependence on the substance or activity that caused the alteration.

Most Diets Don't Work*

Many people battle weight problems.

Just one in every 100 people who go on a diet succeed in shedding weight permanently.

However, the high chance of failure did not stop 34 million Britons trying to lose weight last year, spending more than 10 billion pounds in the process.
....

Lawrence Gould, analyst at Data-monitor, said: "In 2002, 230.6 million people across Europe attempted a diet. Of these, only 3.8 million will succeed in keeping off the weight that they have lost for over a year.

*BBC News, February 19, 2003

Characteristics of addiction include an altered state—a change in clarity or mood when the addictive substance is used, withdrawal if the substance is removed, and relief if it is re-introduced. Addicts will continue to use despite serious threats, negative consequences, and severe losses.

We tend to take food addiction lightly, as if it isn't as difficult as the "hard" addictions. But, really, if it were so easy, how come people can't stay on diets, how come we need ten new diets every year, how come the rate of diet failure is so high? How come 64% of adult Americans are either overweight or obese?[xx]

It's not exactly breaking news that extra weight is bad for you. With serious threats on the horizon such as diabetes, heart disease, joint problems, and limited lifestyle choices, and death rates from obesity nearly doubling in the last 20 years, we've got some good reasons for changing eating.

And most people try. Most overweight people do think they should be helping themselves. They try eating differently, and then slip out of it. Why? Why can't they sustain it?

Because they are actually addicted to certain foods and don't know it. They try to hold on to a new eating plan with willpower and fingernails and it screeches away. Without realizing it, they've run into withdrawal, and under that internal chemical pressure, they return to the old ways of eating.

Body as Commodity Diet, Inc.*

Despite their financial success, commercial diets like [popular diet program] often don't meet their promises.

Diet failure rates hover between 90 and 95 percent, according to Jeanine Cogan, a congressional science fellow for the American Psychological Association. But many of the major companies don't disclose their statistics on success.

*//nm-server.jrn.columbia. edu/projects/masters/ bodyimage/commodity/ index.html

So what is a food addict actually addicted to?

She is addicted to the chemicals that flood her brain when she eats certain foods, and she is addicted to any foods that trigger the flow of those chemicals.

The beauty of food addiction is that it comes in so many varieties. Most food addicts are addicted to sugar, carbohydrates, and fat, but some are specialists, addicted to one but not the others. We have a special subset of chocolate addicts and then there are those who will binge on any food.

We don't have all the brain chain reactions figured out, mainly because there's been so little research. (I think a national epidemic deserves funding for the true cause of the problem, but that's me.)

Here's what we know. There are two areas of (primarily) animal research that point to mechanisms for food addiction. These are the dopamine pathways and the internal opiate system.

Dopamine—the pleasure neurotransmitter

Dopamine is a neurotransmitter. Dopamine neurons are especially plentiful in the limbic system, deep in the center of the brain in areas that have to do with emotion, memory, and sense of smell.

Some researchers wondered if sensitivity to reward, which operates through the dopamine system, would be connected with overeating.

"Sensitivity to reward (STR)—a personality trait firmly rooted in the neurobiology of the mesolimbic dopamine system—has been strongly implicated in the risk for addiction. This construct describes the ability to derive pleasure or reward from natural reinforcers like food, and from pharmacologic rewards like addictive drugs. Recently experts in the field of addiction research have acknowledged that psychomotor stimulant drugs are no longer at the heart of all addictions, and that brain circuits can also be deranged with natural rewards like food." (C. Davis, "Sensitivity to Reward." *Appetite*, 2004.)[xxi]

The Davis study tested whether sensitivity to reward related positively toward overeating and to being overweight, with women of ages 25-45. Indeed, overweight women were far more sensitive to reward than those of normal weight and their overeating correlated positively with their sensitivity. In other words, increased sensitivity to reward was connected to increased eating.

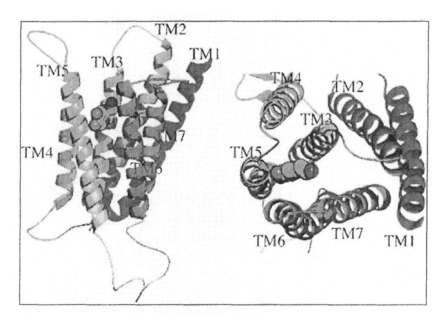

Brain Chemistry 401: The dopamine D2 receptor even looks jolly with its carnival corkscrews. The spheres are dopamine. (Source: Kalani, 2004)

These excellent researchers also found something they weren't looking for. They discovered that women with extra weight tested as more anhedonic and that the degree of extra weight correlated with the degree of being anhedonic.

Anhedonism is a problem with experiencing pleasure. Some of us derive tremendous pleasure from simple things— such as a child's giggle or a snuggling cat or a stroll down a daisy-dappled path—and for others, those same events would make no impression or even, possibly, be irritating.

What could cause this and what does this cause? One very likely cause of anhedonism could be a problem with dopamine functioning.

Some bodies may be set up to become addicted due to a flaw in the dopamine system. Positron Emission Tomography showed that drug addicts had a reduced number of dopamine D2 receptors and that obese subjects showed a similar D2 receptor shortage. In fact, the fewer D2 receptors, the greater body mass index.[xxii]

It makes sense that if your body is naturally deficient in self-soothing, you'd have to juice the system some other way. To make those neurotransmitters flow, find your drug of choice.

Alcoholics find the fastest relief in a bottle. Overeaters will find better relief through eating. Eating, especially sweet eating, activates the dopamine system, as do all the drugs of abuse such as heroin, alcohol, cocaine, amphetamine, as well as nicotine[xxiii] and gambling.[xxiv]

Are Addicts Born or Made?

Both. Let's take each fact of this and the previous chapters, and see how they go together, starting with a person with no genetic pre-disposition toward addiction.

(But first, two additional facts are necessary to understand the following charts. Childhood stress, abuse, neglect, or emotional abandonment cause the formation of neural nets (neuron firing patterns) organized around trauma. These use up two chemicals like a giant sump pump: serotonin—in the search for relief, and norepinephrine [NE].

NE is used in prodigious quantities when we are stressed or frightened. It is also produced when we try hard.)

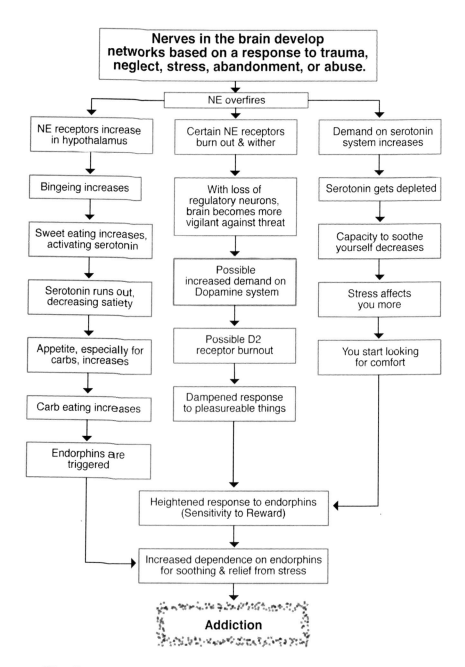

The Development of Food Addiction—Pre-disposition to Addiction Absent

In the Genes

What genetic pre-disposition could increase the risk of becoming addicted to something? Being born with:

- Decreased numbers of D2 dopamine receptors with commensurate flattened response to ordinary pleasures until stumbling upon the delightful hit that comes from consuming candy or some other endorphin promoter like alcohol, drugs, or a compulsive activity.
- Flaws in serotonin functioning, causing heightened sensitivity and vulnerability to stress.

Either condition creates a gateway to the path of addiction.

As you can see, faulty serotonin delivery, within a few steps, leads into the series of physiological events that culminate in addiction. In this way, a person can be pre-disposed to become an addict.

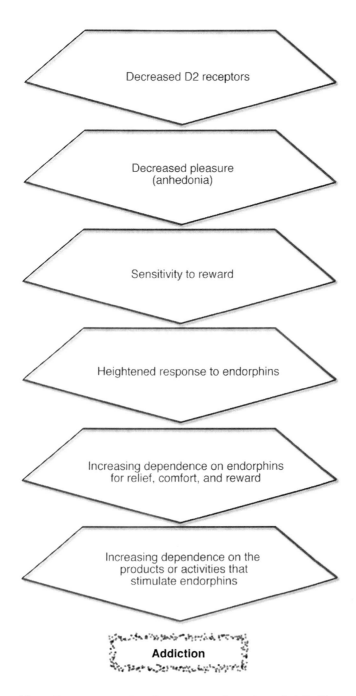

Decreased D2 receptors

Decreased pleasure
(anhedonia)

Sensitivity to reward

Heightened response to endorphins

Increasing dependence on endorphins
for relief, comfort, and reward

Increasing dependence on the
products or activities that
stimulate endorphins

Addiction

How Decreased D2 Receptors Lead to Addiction

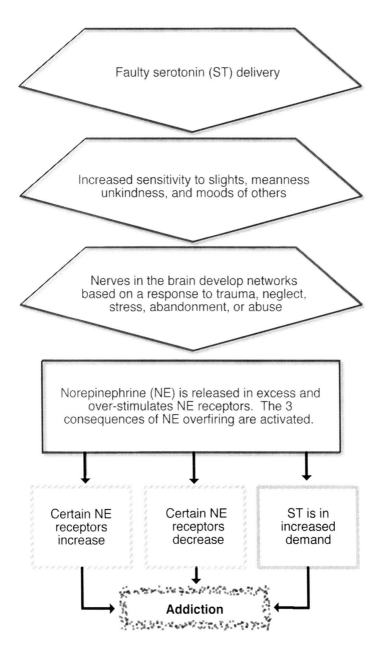

How Faulty Serotonin Delivery Leads to Addiction

Food addiction is a real condition

It's not only as serious as any other addiction, causing cascading losses in both health and quality of life, it has a built-in major league snag. Food addicts can't give up food.

Alcoholics, smokers, and junkies can become abstinent and never consume their substance again. They can stay away from the people and places that are associated with using. There's very little reason for an alcoholic to ever re-enter a bar or a smoker to ever hold a cigarette in his hands. Ever.

Not ever, do these addicts have to get up close and personal with their substance.

Off the top of your head, can you identify five ways this situation is different for food addicts?

How is food addiction recovery more difficult than recovery from other substance addictions:

1.
2.
3.
4.
5.

Here are the ones I came up with. Food addicts:

1. Encounter their substance daily
2. Handle their substance frequently
3. Are surrounded by their substance whenever they have to grocery shop
4. Must actually take their substance into their mouths daily
5. Encounter their substance at all sorts of venues that are not actual eating places
6. Are surrounded by people freely consuming their substance

Do:

- Open your mind to an acceptance of food addiction as a real condition.
- Look at the chain reactions that lead to food addiction a couple of times so that you are familiar with the factors involved. You don't have to memorize them.

If you are interested in the actual physiology of food addiction—the parts of the brain, the sequence of physiological events—that description is in *How to Make Almost Any Diet Work*, chapter 17.

Would you be willing to experience an allegory that puts you in the chair of a person with these struggles? Please read the following excerpt from *How to Make Almost Any Diet Work*. (Otherwise, skip to the next chapter.)

Sit Down with the Dragon[xxv]

The family drew near the old farmhouse in high spirits. Before Uncle Harry even pushed his car door shut, Papa Blaine called quips from the porch. Joan reached down to help her sister Gloria lug a huge basket of exotic fare up the porch steps. Meanwhile, Aunt Barbara leaned out of the doorway to wave people indoors, admitting a few bright leaves as well. They skittered along the polished floor, and Cousin Milli grabbed them for the centerpiece.

Three people—Grandma, Caroline, and Gerald—faced this event with anxiety. Grandma was fighting a battle with diabetes—and the sugary foods she could no longer have; Caroline had started and stopped more times than she wanted to count; and Gerald had been in solid recovery for five years. They'd have been better off not attending, but this autumn tradition was an important family event, and they didn't want to miss a chance to be with people they loved.

Finally, all was ready and the whole crowd gathered at the large oak table. Everyone took a seat and, one by one, each selection was passed around.

Grandpa introduced his gift first. "This is a perky little cabernet I found in the Robe Valley. It's from a small family vineyard that doesn't even have a label, but I pried this out of them. It's as smooth as syrup. Everyone have a taste."

Grandma, wanting to show support for her husband, lifted the wineglass to her lips and took a small sip. Caroline pretended to sip and tried not to inhale the full-bodied scent of the wine. The three glasses in front of Gerald stayed empty; he planned to drink coffee.

Papa Blaine bounced to his feet. "Listen, everybody, I can't wait. You've got to try mine next. It looks just like an ordinary claret but it's much more."

Cousin Ed protested, "No, no. Try these instead." He gestured to his wife who began passing a fancy bowl filled with orange capsules. "I found these at a little market in Colombia. Take these and the rest of the day will be unbelievably vivid."

Linda, just back from her first year at college, interrupted, "Try my pot first. It's the favorite of everyone on campus."

Great-Grandma's authoritative wheeze cut through the chaos. "Now children, you know we drink the wines first, before we have the pills and pot."

Everyone subsided with little murmurs of apology.

Grandma watched as Grandpa filled her row of glasses with each new wine that came by. How was she going to get through this day without drinking? No matter how many times she tried to explain to her husband that she was an alcoholic, he didn't seem to get it. True to form he continued to describe each new wine glowingly, wanting her to have a taste of each one.

Caroline had been sober just three months. She looked at her filled wine-glasses, thinking she wasn't going to get through this afternoon with her sobriety intact. She didn't want to seem different or call attention to herself. She wished she could be like the others who could drink all these wines and then just stop, but she knew that if she had even a little bit, she'd fall back into a non-stop binge.

Gerald gritted his teeth and sipped his coffee. Years of solid recovery didn't protect him from the scent of the wine. Although he jovially passed each bottle, joining in with the jokes and laughter, this get-together was not easy for him. He used to be a secret drinker, so he knew the most dangerous time for him would be after the event, during clean-up, when his relatives' backs were turned and he was tempted to pick up their glasses and swallow the little mouthfuls of wine that remained.

19
Trigger and Drug Foods

Curious?
What is a trigger food?
What is a drug food?
If you take over, will she do better?

She's addicted to the brain chemicals that reward her, and she's addicted to the foods that have the power to stimulate those chemicals. Her task will be to identify which foods have that power.

Trigger foods are those foods which trigger her to eat more. Some foods are pistol triggers—when consumed, they trigger a person to eat more of the same item. Peanut butter is a pistol trigger food for some people. When they eat one spoonful of peanut butter, they want more and more peanut butter, but no other foods.

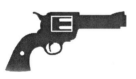

Peanut butter is a common pistol trigger.

Peanut Butter Pistol Trigger

Shotgun triggers stimulate increased eating across the board. Sugar is such a food for many people. When they have sugar, not only do they eat more sugary things, but their eating spreads out, including starchy, salty, and fatty foods, and larger portion sizes even of proteins and of ordinary meal items.

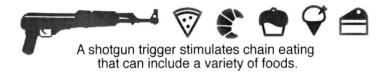

A shotgun trigger stimulates chain eating
that can include a variety of foods.

Shotgun Triggers Shoot Trouble

Drug foods are those foods which alter mood or consciousness. Such foods are capable of stimulating the addictive pathways in the brain. Trigger and drug foods can be the same foods.

For most, but not all, people, sugar is a powerful trigger food *and* it alters mood and consciousness. Other good candidates are breads, fried food, refined starches, most wheat products, soft drinks, ice cream, chocolate, and high fat foods, such as sour cream, mayonnaise, butter, and cream.

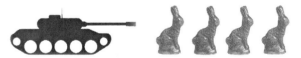

Chocolate brings out the big guns.

Chocolate—Major Drug Food

Sometimes, when a person gets rid of her major trigger foods, she can tolerate small amounts of marginal foods without being triggered. For example, when someone has a solid abstinence from sugar, bread, and wheat, she may be able to eat wraps without being triggered or losing abstinence.

She'll have to go through her own process of identifying her drug and trigger foods, and you can't help her with this. This is something she has to do with her recovery partner.

Most food addicts have to struggle to develop an honest list. In part, revealing her trigger foods—even to her recovery partner— takes her eating out of the closet. She can feel as if she's giving up control of her primary source of relief and comfort. She may fear that someone will misuse the list and start micromanaging her eating. She may well feel shame at revealing just how important some foods are.

To disclose these foods takes a lot of courage and tremendous trust. She'll have a much better chance at making an honest list if she does this first with her recovery partner and support group.

In fact, don't even ask. Don't ask what her trigger foods are. Don't ask where she is in the process of identifying them. And, by all means, don't tell her what you think are her trigger foods.

Do:

- Refrain from telling her what her drug and trigger foods are.

Don't:

- Don't ask.
- Don't tell.

When she starts abstinence, she'll have to let you know what foods are persona non grata. By sharing her list with you, she'll be investing you with great trust. Here's how to stay worthy of it:

Leave authority over her program in her hands.

20

Abstinence

An addict gets clean and an alcoholic gets sober. This means they refrain completely from any use of their substance. An alcoholic abstains from all forms of alcohol—whiskey, wine, brandy, beer, and hard cider.

For food addicts, the equivalent to being clean and sober is abstinence. But, of course, it's more complicated. As much as they wish they could, they cannot abstain from all food. They have to define their abstinence, based not only on what food groups trigger them, but also on the specific items within each food group that trigger them.

Certain foods, and certain forms of food, require complete and total abstinence. This means none, nada, not ever, not for any reason. Other foods won't trigger them if kept to certain quantities and eaten in certain contexts.

Let's take rice as an example. Some people have an addictive reaction to white rice, and a relatively small serving will be a shotgun trigger, stimulating them to add butter and gravy or sugar, raisins, and cinnamon. From here they may move on to nuts, popcorn, or some sort of bread or pastry.

Brown rice, in limited quantities, in the context of a meal with plenty of protein, may not be a trigger. They can eat a half cup of rice seasoned with herbs and garlic, after they've had their broccoli and pork chop, and leave the table looking forward to a sudoku puzzle.

For this reason, no one can have a perfect abstinence right out of the chute. This will be a trial and error process. As their systems get cleaner, they'll start to notice that dip in alertness or energy that signals a drugged state, or the sneaky return of a craving after eating a particular food.

An alcoholic can get abstinent from all forms of alcohol at once. But food addicts, unless they are in a treatment center, may not be able to achieve total abstinence of all drug and trigger foods on their first try.

Some folks have a greater chance at success if they abstain from one major shotgun trigger at a time, refining their food plan gradually. As they get comfortable with abstinence from one food group, they are then able to tackle the next food group. Achieving their optimal abstinence can take more than a year, and even then, as their bodies weather various changes in hormones, wellness, and activity level, their abstinence will require re-tooling.

It's an intensely personal process, and you will be walking a very fine line. Please continue.

21

Your Delicate Position

Curious?
Will it work to monitor her eating?
Should you watch with disapproval when she eats?
Is it OK to eat her trigger foods in front of her?

You inhabit a powerful position in relation to the food addict you love. You can offer the timely support that solidifies her recovery, or you can add the last straw that breaks its back.

Here's an example. Let's suppose she now realizes that she is indeed a food addict, and she is in the final stages of preparing for abstinence. Question: Which of the following actions will sabotage her?

1. "Honey, since you're planning to give up sugar on Monday, let's go out for one last sugar blast."
2. "Honey, you are going to have to give up sugar forever."

(Answer: *Both statements can sabotage her.*)

I'm going to make an unequivocal statement. Your challenge is to use this information properly, without making it into a hammer that will damage her progress.

Here goes:

If she is a food addict, she will have to become abstinent from her drug and shotgun trigger foods if she is to have lasting relief from her appetite disorder.

How you use this information matters a lot. Your job is to walk the delicate line of offering support without triggering her defiance or resistance.

Here are the actions that will backfire, and that risk cata-
pulting her back into her addiction.

Don't:

- Don't tell her what she can't eat.
- Don't monitor her eating.
- Don't control her eating or her access to food.
- Don't check up on the kitchen supplies to see what she
  has eaten.
- Don't watch with disapproval as she eats.
- Don't criticize or judge her eating.
- Don't call her names when she eats.

I guarantee that if you try to control her, she will, outside of
your presence, eat even more of her drug foods than if you hadn't
interfered. And she will only become more clandestine in her eating. Is this what you want?

Secret eating breeds the shame cycle and leads to more eating to numb the shame. It fans the flames of the addiction.

So, controlling her is out. Inside, she'll say to herself, "You
can't control me!" and eat whatever her addiction wants.

What you *can* do is provide alternatives to her drug foods,
and take care about what foods you expose her to.

* * *

The following *Do and Don't* lists are the most important in
this book. The very best and most powerful support springs from
these principles.

Do Reduce Her Exposure to Drug and Trigger Foods

- Support her in removing her drug and trigger foods from
  her home.
  - ❍ Help her box them up.
  - ❍ Transport them to a place that can use them.
  - ❍ If you live with her, establish a separate place for the
    foods you like that aren't on her "safe to eat" list. (A
    cabinet, closet, or drawer she never has any reason
    to open are examples.)

Don't Expose her to her drug or trigger foods.
- Don't eat her drug or trigger foods in front of her.
  - ○ Be thoughtful about not eating desserts, pastries, breads, sandwiches, pancakes, French toast, syrup, etc. in front of her. *Remember, you can have these foods anywhere you want, whenever you want. You don't have to deprive yourself. Just don't eat them in front of her.*
  - ○ Don't leave plates with crumbs, syrup, melted sauce, butter, or ice cream for her to clean up.
  - ○ Don't leave a half eaten dessert on the kitchen counter for her to put away.
  - ○ Don't leave bags of cookies, candies, chips, or crackers—open or closed—lying around for her to find.
  - ○ Don't leave candy or pastry wrappers in the car.
  - ○ Don't leave candy bits on the seat or floor of the car.
  - ○ Don't ask her to prepare her drug or trigger foods, not even for a good cause.
  - ○ Don't volunteer her cookies for the office party unless you plan to bake them yourself when she isn't home.
  - ○ Don't ask her to make her famous strudel for the church breakfast.
  - ○ Don't expect her to make your favorite cake for your birthday. Ask her for the recipe and let your sister, cousin, or buddy make it for you. (Or make it yourself when she won't be home for awhile.)
  - ○ Help her revise the menu for traditional meals so that there's a version of every main dish for her. An alternative Thanksgiving menu appears in the Appendix of this book.

You already know that …

The American culture is deluged with food. It is a major part of most events. We're used to having all sorts of tempting food nearly everywhere we go. So how illogical is it to expect a food addict to resist food if she is constantly bombarded with it?

I play bridge once a week, and my club's tradition is to serve sweet snacks and a dessert. For years, my abstinence would hold up until I got to bridge night. Over and over I fell off the wagon as I sat with a bowl of sweets two inches from my hand.

At first I tried to resist it. But exposure to food reduces satiety and increases appetite. Willpower cannot defeat brain chemistry.

Finally, a friend in my recovery group said, "Take something you can eat."

At the time, I felt childish about needing to have my own little treat, but finally I surrendered and took my own food to every bridge night. I made a point to take something delicious but safe: fresh pineapple chunks, strawberries, almonds, frozen grapes (that the host allowed me to tuck into a freezer).

When the hostess served dessert, I pulled out my treat and ate it. The result was magical. I no longer felt deprived or different. I not only enjoyed my treat, but noticed that after the snack, some of the others played worse bridge, while I stayed alert.

Now, whenever I go into an eating situation where I know temptations will abound, I take my own treat. It works wonderfully.

Do Provide Foods She Can Eat

There are three ways you can support the person you love:
- Encourage her to take or bring her own food.
  - Suggest that she take her own treats when she'll be going somewhere with tempting food.
  - Encourage her to take an abstinent food she'll enjoy if she's going to a potluck (so that she's guaranteed that there'll be something she can eat).
- Provide options that are on her food plan.
  - Make a sugar-free dessert so that she'll have something special while others are eating their sweets. (Check with her to see what sugar-free products work for her. Even some sugar-free products can be dangerous for her.)
  - If you're serving an entrée that she doesn't eat, such as pasta, provide another entrée for her, such as brown rice that she can dress with red sauce and cheese.

◯ If you are providing snacks, have at least one snack or appetizer she can eat, such as stuffed celery, olives, marinated artichoke hearts, nuts, or cheese cubes.

◯ Don't dish up plates. Let guests serve themselves.

◯ If you aren't sure what's on her food plan, it's a great kindness to check with her while you're still planning your menu.

◯ Make it easy for her to leave the table early. When I'm in a situation where everyone is oohing over a fancy, aromatic dessert, I have to leave the table and the room. She, too, will have to guard her sight and smell neurons by making a fast and strategic retreat from the table. You can support her by giving her something to do or to look at. ("Honey, go look at the new book I got. It's on the table in the family room," or "Would you mind watering the roses?")

22

Withdrawal

Curious?
Do dieters go through withdrawal?
Should she make an important decision while she's in withdrawal?
How long does withdrawal last?

She tried to read. Normally she was a fast and focused reader, but every few minutes a craving waved across her body, clenching her insides. She'd ride it out like a birthing pain, or grief, and every time, as it peaked, she thought she surely couldn't bear it. Then it would drop off so fast it was as if it had never been.

She returned to her book. But the picture of a drive-through soon formed in her head. She could almost smell the French fries. She wanted it. She wanted it. She'd get in her car right now and drive to one if she hadn't brought herself to this island that didn't have a single drive-through or restaurant.

Finally, after four hours of desperate cravings, it was time to walk to the dining hall. She was halfway there when she realized that she'd forgotten to bring her ticket. As she turned to go back to her room, she thought, *Why am I doing this? I could get in my car, be at the ferry in thirty minutes, and be at a restaurant two hours from now.*

The idea had such substance that as she entered her room, she lifted her suitcase and opened it. Then she stood there, looking blankly through the window at the pulsing sea. If she left now, she would return to the craziness of hating her body, guilt about eating, thinking constantly of food, and planning ways to get away from her family so she could eat. If she left now, she'd be miserable, a different miserable, one that wouldn't ever stop. If she stayed, she'd only be really miserable for another few days.

She turned and left the room, halfway to the lodge before remembering that she still didn't have her ticket.

As she pivoted, a woman she'd tried to befriend walked by without a word. Rage flashed through her. Her mind filled with seventeen ways to punish her. She concocted a devilish passive-aggressive plot. Then she felt despair, rejection. She wasn't good enough. An aloneness hollowed her so deeply, she couldn't catch a breath.

Back at her room, she wanted to collapse on her bed, but a glance at the clock told her she had 20 minutes before the dining room would close its doors. She grabbed her ticket and ran.

If anyone doubts the reality of food addiction, they need only witness or experience withdrawal. Being hounded by cravings, disturbances of mind, disorientation—attends withdrawal from food addiction just as it does withdrawal from alcohol or other drugs.

Withdrawal is signaled by one or more of the following:

- Strong cravings and substance-seeking behavior
- Irritation, rage, impatience, or anger if someone or something gets in the way as she heads toward her substance
- Willingness to cross ethical or moral boundaries to obtain the substance even if it causes hurt or deprivation for a loved one
- Manipulation of people or a situation in order to obtain the substance
- Distorted thinking

Withdrawal is what defeats dieters. Without realizing it, the confusion and cravings caused by endorphin withdrawal push them to cheat on their diets. Then, once they've consumed their drug food, the joyful rush of addictive brain chemicals pulls them back into the addictive trap.

For an alcoholic, a hangover is the start of withdrawal. Similarly, every time a food addict is removed for too long from her substance, she will experience withdrawal. Then, a part of her will be focused on obtaining her drug food, no matter how well she screens this by appearing to function normally.

She herself may not be consciously aware that while blazing away at the computer another part of her mind is mapping the route to the sweet store. It can control her, even if she isn't conscious of how her brain is directing her. It can cause her to mislead others, mislead herself, and defy her most fervent commitments around eating.

One of the fruits of abstinence is clear thinking. Once she is abstinent, her brain won't be able to trick her so quietly. The longer she is abstinent, the more she'll be able to catch the traps set by the cunning addicted brain.

But getting there is tough. And the only way to cross the river to the land of sobriety is to navigate the waters of withdrawal.

You can be a huge help. First, understand the symptoms of withdrawal.

Symptoms of Withdrawal

Withdrawal is a sign that the addicted part of the brain is having a tantrum. Like a little kid kicking and screaming in the checkout line, those receptor cells are yearning for their treat. Neurons that were used to the soothing wash of endorphins are gonna buzz. They'll be super sensitive for awhile and likely to overreact. This will manifest in some combination of the following symptoms:

- Strong, sneaky cravings that may or may not be easily identified as cravings
- Ideas or thoughts that position her near trigger or drug foods
- Strong feeling of wanting or needing something that is missing
- Disorientation
- Loss of perspective
- Forgetfulness
- Irritability
- Disturbed sleep
- Anxiety
- Aches and pains
- Confusion
- Heightened startle response
- Mood swings

- Weepy
- Loss of insight as to the reason for the discomfort or disturbances
- Amnesia about why the heck she's feeling so unlike herself

How You Can Help

You can give some seriously important help to your loved one during this time. You'll continue to see the big picture while she's totally lost her signal.

Do:

Help her remember the reason for her discomfort. Though it seems patently obvious, she'll actually forget that there's a name for what she's going through and that it's called withdrawal. She'll even forget that it's connected to liberating herself from her drug foods.

Remind her that this will pass. Having lost her perspective, she'll feel as if this confusion and disorientation will go on forever. Remind her that within days this will start to clear up.

Help her to stay on her program. Remind her to have her snacks. Encourage her to call her recovery partner.

Give her turkey. She'll really be needing tryptophan during this time. It will help many of her symptoms. If she doesn't eat turkey, encourage her to have whatever she substitutes for it. She should be eating a good source of tryptophan every day the first week of abstinence.

Give her grapefruit. (Not juice, but the whole fruit). For some reason, it helps with withdrawal.

Don't worry about portion sizes. She may overeat other foods, trying to get a fix from them. If she's still eating some of her drug foods, this may work. If she's abstaining from all her major drug foods at once, this won't work.

A common thought of food addicts in withdrawal is, "Since I'm overeating even worse this week, I might as well eat my drug food again." This is so illogical, I don't know where to start, but these are the kind of thoughts an addicted brain has.

Provide the voice of reason with a rebuttal such as, "Honey, honor your commitment to yourself. If you'll stick with this a few more days, your eating will begin to normalize."

Help her stay in the moment. The phrase, 'one day at a time,' may seem like a cliché, but it comes into its own during withdrawal. She'll have thoughts like, "I'll never get to have this again. I can't stand to go my whole life without another _____."

Say things like, "Sweetie, you only have to let go of that food today. Can you get through the next moment without that food?"

Stand by with spare keys. Be willing to rescue her if she locks her keys in the car, loses her keys to the house, can't find her calendar. These things will happen during the firestorm of withdrawal.

Encourage her to wait to make any important decisions. She won't be able to think clearly enough to make good decisions this week.

Being a Super Hero

Take over providing meals this week. Asking a food addict to prepare meals her first week of abstinence is like making an alcoholic bartend during his first week of sobriety. It's truly not fair.

Good, healthy meals can be had, even at fast food places: salads, roasted chicken, turkey burger—hold the bun. Asian take-out (no msg), those roasted chickens provided by large supermarkets, vegetable trays—it can be easy to find prepared abstinent foods so that she doesn't have to shop or visit a drive-through.

Have the family fix their own lunches. Give her a break from kitchen duty.

Rinse any plates or dishes you're leaving for her to wash. Protect her from encountering crumbs or other tempting scraps.

How Long Does It Last?

The physical consequences of withdrawal last for about three weeks, but the intensity falls off sharply after the first week. She'll feel remarkably better by her second week, and even a little cocky, but it's not time yet to rest on laurels. Withdrawal will reappear now and then, diminishing in strength over time.

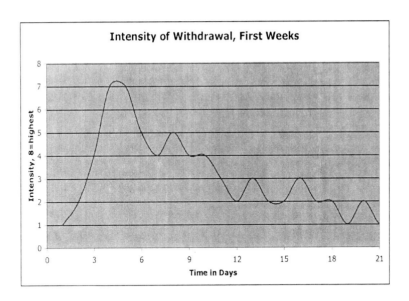

Not everyone will follow this same pattern. If she's abstaining from all her trigger foods at once, withdrawal will hit sooner, harder, and last longer. On the other hand, once she's past the first intense period—two to four weeks—she'll be surprised at her deliverance from cravings and how clear her mind is.

Occasionally, someone has an easy withdrawal. This gift is a rare one, and it carries the danger that she won't treasure her abstinence. If the addicted brain starts seducing her with thoughts like, "You didn't go through withdrawal, so you're not really addicted," she may fall back into addictive eating. The odds are, if she goes for abstinence again at a later time, withdrawal will be brutal.

After the first month, it starts getting a lot easier to stay abstinent. During this time, it's tempting to get sloppy on support and snacking. But it's important for everyone to remember that this reprieve from the addiction comes to you courtesy of satiety and surrender. The addition is a sleeping dragon. It wakes easily. It pounces fast.

For some reason, there are certain anniversaries after one's first abstinence at which cravings and addictive thoughts resurge. These occur around 90, 180, and 270 days after her first abstinence.

Each yearly anniversary is also a time that the dragon looks around to see if he can sneak back in. The major eating holidays activate appetite as well.

The following chart shows these surges plotted over a time period of 13 months. Her surges could be higher or lower at any given point. (And one more surge would occur—from Thanksgiving through New Year's Day, wherever that would fall on her first year of abstinence.)

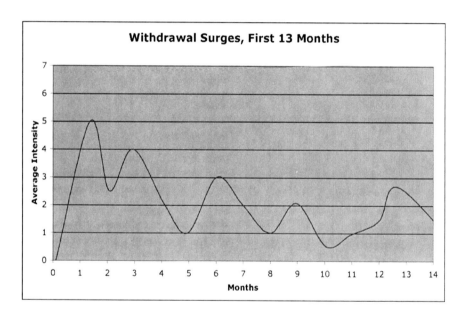

Even after a year of abstinence, there will be a resurgence of vulnerability to the dragon. The diciest times will be periods of high stress and yearly anniversaries. As always, when stress goes up, she will be most successful if she increases her tryptophan intake. (She knows all about appropriate sources of tryptophan from her book or program.)

Do:

- Celebrate her abstinence birthday with a card and a hurrah. You will help her realize just how far she's come.
- This is really the time to protect her from idiots who say, "One bite won't hurt."

23

Perfect Abstinence

No such thing. Her abstinence will be a process of refinement. And we all have to get over the wish that it can be as clear and defined as it is for alcoholics and other drug addicts.

It you're alcoholic, it's alcohol, period. AA meetings celebrate annual sobriety birthdays (often with cake) and to earn that yearly coin, an alcoholic has to be alcohol-free for the duration of the period recognized. If he gets a 21-year coin, he has to be free of all forms of alcohol for the entire 21 years.

Such a stringent requirement actually messes up abstinence for many food addicts. They tell themselves, or others say, that if they have a mere crust, their previous days of abstinence no longer count. I've seen too many people lose recovery from the pervading sense of failure that comes from believing that with every new try they are starting from scratch.

Food addiction recovery is a complicated process. For one thing, each person's abstinence has to be personally defined. If you are triggered by chick peas and I'm not, you'll have to back off chick peas and I don't. For another, the list of triggering foods actually shifts with age, hormones, and lifestyle.

The three main problems that occur with first abstinence are these:

- Making abstinence too strict. Food addicts can be self-punitive and believe that they have to restrict themselves from all foods they enjoy. This can set them up to get bored with their food plan and rebel against its narrowness.

- Making abstinence too loose. Out of fear of facing the world unshielded, food addicts can leave holes in their abstinence large enough to drive a binge through. Signs that the abstinence boundaries need to be tightened include:
  - ◯ Continued overeating
  - ◯ Continued focus on obtaining and consuming food
  - ◯ Ongoing cravings past the normal end of the withdrawal period
- Following someone else's abstinence. Certain food addiction recovery programs dictate the abstinence their members are to follow. The problem with this is that one plan does not fit all. We all have different chemistries. If I try to stay abstinent from foods that don't trigger me, I will eventually resent it and rebel, with the risk of ditching my entire abstinence instead of simply taking that one item off the abstinence list.

What This Means for Her

She'll do best if she continues to work with her recovery partner and her support group (if she participates in a recovery program) or a 12-step group. There, she can be honest about what foods are still triggering her and about black and white thoughts that push her toward depriving herself.

And Birthdays

I say celebrate the birthday of the first abstinence as long as she is staying connected to recovery. Food addicts slip. It's part of the disease. Rather than make a slip a big deal, leading to a loss of all abstinence, she can be cleanly abstinent again right now. Today, she is abstinent again, and can climb back on her plan and call her partner or go to a meeting.

What This Means for You

- You can't superintend her abstinence process. If you try to monitor her abstinence or the foods she's choosing, you risk sparking her defiance and secrecy.

- If she seems to be setting herself up with either two strict or too loose an abstinence, encourage her to talk to her recovery partner about it.
- You may have a slight bit of influence at getting her to loosen a too strict plan, but frankly, as a food addiction therapist with years of experience, I say, "Good luck with that." When I have a client setting herself up this way, all I can do is give a light sketch of the possible consequences and leave the choice with her. In thirty years of specializing in food addiction, I've never been able to get a client to relax a too-strict plan for abstinence. They have to go through the consequences, and then they can start over with a more moderate plan.
- Cultivate a light-hearted detachment from her food choices.

I know this is very hard to do. I love someone who is dying from obesity and for years I tried every arrow in my sling to promote recovery for her. Eventually I had to let it go. I love her. And she gets to make her own choices. I went through all the stages of grief, and came finally to acceptance. So, finally, I pay no attention to her food and savor, instead, the moments I share with her.

You can get there too. Read chapter 26 or go to an O-Anon meeting. (Like Al-Anon, but for people who love an overeater. Since these meetings are scarce, you can also find help at an Al-Anon meeting, many of which now recognize that regardless of the type of addiction, loved ones need their own program.)

24

The Top Thirteen Things To Never Say

Absolutely, Positively Never Say:

1. "Just one bite won't hurt."
2. "Just have a taste."
3. "Keep me company while I eat dessert."
4. "I don't want to eat my ice cream alone. Join me."
5. "Honey, hand me the cookies."
6. "I got these special diet pills for you off the internet."
7. "Mmmm, this is the best lemon pie I've ever had."
8. "If I can't give you chocolate for Valentine's Day (Christmas, your birthday), what can I give you?" (Stated in a whiny tone of voice.)
9. "I heard about this new diet. Edna lost 30 pounds in two weeks. I think you should try it."
10. "If you love me, you'll make those special cookies for me."
11. "If I don't have your coconut cake, it won't feel like my birthday."
12. "If you gain any more weight:
    a. Your husband will leave you."
    b. You'll lose your job."
    c. I can't be friends anymore."
    d. Your clothes won't fit."
    e. You'll be ashamed to go anywhere."
    f. My friends will think I'm a bad mother."
    g. You won't fit on an airplane."
    h. It will reflect on me."
    i. The planets will shift in their orbits."
13. "Why not just have the surgery?"

Exercise Your Smart Muscles

Now that you're educated about appetite disorder and food addiction, I bet you can give the reason for refraining from these sabotaging statements. (Give it a try if you want to test yourself, then check your ideas against my responses in the following list.)

In case you do need quick rebuttals the next time you protect her from the ignorance of Aunt Clueless or Uncle Whiney, here they are:

1. "Just one bite won't hurt."
   It will, actually. One bite of a triggering food can cause a relapse.

2. "Just have a taste."
   Please stop tempting her. It isn't kind since one bite of a triggering food can cause a relapse.

3. "Keep me company while I eat dessert."
   The sight and smell of a tempting food will increase her appetite and risk relapse.

4. "I don't want to eat my ice cream alone. Join me."
   Uncle Whiney, please stop increasing her exposure to sweet foods. That will only increase her appetite chemicals and make her eat more stuff.

5. "Honey, hand me the cookies."
   Aunt Clueless, I'll get the cookies for you. Please don't ask her to put herself in harm's way. Contact with tempting food will increase her appetite chemicals and can cause a relapse.

6. "Mmmm, this is the best lemon pie I've ever had. It is so creamy."
   Aunt Clueless, it would be kind to savor it quietly. Comments that make the forbidden fruit even more vivid, increase the pull toward the food. Also, if she feels left out or deprived, keeping abstinent is harder.

7. "I got these special diet pills for you off the internet."
   Diet pills always backfire. They either cause rebound appetite, promote addiction to the pills themselves, or cause other types of damage. They can seduce her into believing she can eat whatever she wants without consequences.

8. "If I can't give you chocolate for Valentine's Day (Christmas, your birthday), what can I give you?" (Stated in a whiny tone of voice.)
    (This is a plea for her to return to her old persona, the one who doesn't take care of herself and sacrifices herself for others.) Uncle Whiney, remember that a true gift is for the recipient not the giver.

9. "I heard about this new diet. Edna lost 30 pounds in two weeks. I think you should try it."
    Her focus has to stay with her appetite switch. A diet will distract her from what really causes her to eat. (If she has serious support (5 meetings a week), has kept her appetite chemicals balanced for a year, and has been abstinent for two years, she can, very gingerly, try a diet. She should choose a diet based on how it fits her chemical profile. The process for this is in How to Make Almost Any Diet Work. *Once she's chosen her course, it's disruptive for her to switch each time some new wonder comes into view.)*

10. "If you love me, you'll make those cookies for me."
    Aunt Clueless, handling sweets will trigger her appetite and risk a relapse. If you love her, don't ask her to sacrifice her health for you.

11. "If I don't have your coconut cake, it won't feel like my birthday."
    (This is a plea for her to sacrifice her needs for someone else's special occasion.) Uncle Whiney, she'll give you her recipe and you can ask someone else to fix it.

12. "If you gain any more weight...
    Don't threaten her, please. Threats increase norepinephrine which increases appetite and a desire for comfort food. They work against the goal of satiety.

13. "Why not just have the surgery?
    Aunt Clueless, we sometimes long for a quick fix too, but each time there's a new surgical answer to weight loss, it takes time to see what the costs are going to be. The side effects and long-term consequences are sometimes more dangerous or annoying than the original weight. But what is clear is this,

even after surgery, she would still be addicted to food. She would still crave food and she would still want to overeat. Some of these surgeries are not reversible. Once a person has it, she's stuck with the consequences.

25

Stress-Caused Eating

Curious?
How does stress cause eating?
Can stress eating lead to food addiction?
Will it turn out well if you say, "Honey, I notice you're eating more lately?

By sticking up for her in dicey situations, you help reduce the stress that causes comfort eating. You already know all about the relief and soothing that comes from food-triggered endorphins, so it's not surprising that, before abstinence, when she was seeking comfort, she turned to food.

Even after abstinence, stress will increase her appetite and her vulnerability for relapse. The chemical process that makes this happen works through norepinephrine (NE). NE is another neurotransmitter that carries messages from one neuron to another.

The Effort Neurotransmitter

Norepinephrine makes people try hard. Put very simply, serotonin soothes, dopamine dopes, and NE activates. When someone is trying hard, being overactive, busy, fretful, or reactive, then you can imagine that NE is flowing like a river.

But what does this have to do with eating? Way back in Chapter 18, you studied a flow chart that described the chemical steps that lead to addiction. The second step (on page 54) referred to NE over-firing and then becoming depleted and the two streams that proceed from that:

- A brain that has trouble turning itself off
- Physical changes in the eating center

We don't have to go over all that again. What matters is that in the presence of ongoing stress, certain NE receptors are burning out while, in some hypothalamic eating centers, other receptors may actually be increasing or becoming more sensitive.

NE Tsunami

Flooding norepinephrine can cause:

- Glucose intolerance[xxvi]
- Increased triglycerides[xxvii]
- Increased abdominal fat[xxviii]
- Increased weight[xxix]
- Fat production[xxx]
- Increased eating[xxxi][xxxii]
- Insulin resistance
- Impairment of cognitive function[xxxiii]

This means that stress can cause her weigh more, eat more, and store more fat. It can also impair her judgment, thereby disrupting her recovery and her recovery priorities.

In the morning, after she meditates, she may be very clear about her intention to talk to her recovery partner. In the late afternoon, after a hard day at work, she may actually forget her commitment and head for a drive-thru.

As the chemical link between stress and eating is reinforced—and ongoing or long-lasting stress potentiates cellular changes—then sugar and starch are stumbled on as a way to calm the whole system down. As you already know, they do this by, initially, promoting serotonin production and then dopamine activation. Once dopamine pathways are reinforced, she has crossed the bridge to addiction. The circuit is completed and stress will then lead directly to comfort eating and staunch addiction.

These are all excellent reasons to partner her in reducing her stress.

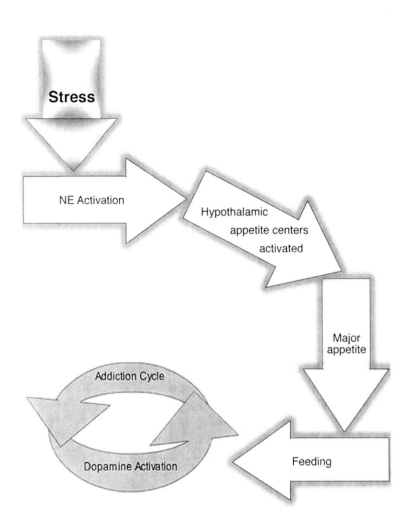

How Stress Leads to Hard-Wired Addiction

Stress Triggers Withdrawal-like Symptoms

    The initial physical effects of withdrawal pass fairly quickly, but it is here, in the reaction to stress, that withdrawal lingers. When she gets stressed, cravings will reappear, and with that

peculiar amnesia around withdrawal and addiction, she won't nec-
essarily be able to link her cravings with the situation that caused
it.

You are in a better position to notice. If you see her browsing the cupboards or making restaurant suggestions that put her in
a slippery place or eating more than usual, then you can deduce
that something is stressing her. In fact any way she is deserting her
program is such a sign—skipping snacks, not using support, eating
marginal foods.

The dragon that is the addiction has awakened. It's raven-
ous. It's setting her up to relapse.

Which of the following comments will promote a return to
recovery?

1. "Honey, I notice you're eating more lately. Are you wor-
    ried about something?"
2. "Daughter, is that a sandwich? I thought you weren't
    supposed to have bread. "
3. "Sweetie, I think something's bothering you. Let's have
    some tea and talk about things in our lives."

Example 1 may sound okay to you, but it will cause trouble.
Remember, she's tottering on the edge of a relapse. If there's any
way to take something wrong, it's gonna happen when she's in this
frame of mind. Any hint that someone is watching what she eats
will put her back up, even on a good day. With this comment, you
risk triggering a reaction along the lines of, "You can't tell me what
to eat. I'll have what I damn well please."

You may be thinking that the second sentence of example 1
demonstrates your concern, but I doubt if she'll even hear it. She'll
be too busy reacting to the first sentence.

Example 2 can also spark defiance. Monitoring someone's
food is experienced as a threat to autonomy and most of the time,
she will react by proving she is in charge, even if that means eating
food that hurts her.

Example 3 is kind and creates an opening. She may be
resistant to noticing what she is feeling, but by constructing a cozy
setting, you are inviting her to calm into herself, which will relax
boundaries and allow for an exchange of information.

You are a safety net. In fact, here is where you come into your own. You had to hang back and step lightly around the abstinence process, but when it comes to offering relief from stress, you are a major player in her life.

Do:

- Create an opening. "Honey, come sit by me and tell me about your day."
- Offer her ways to get healthy relief from stress.
- Practice the skills that help people contain feelings. Next chapter, please.

26

Put Your Feelings into a Bowl

As a child, were you taught to embrace your feelings or to avoid them? Most of us have been trained to avoid feelings, learning to ignore, suppress, or deny them, and even to act them out. Such methods cause feelings to sit undigested in our bodies, getting heavier as more feelings pile up.

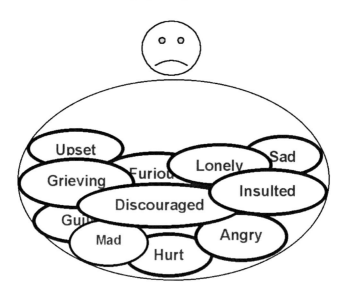

With the passage of time, suppressed feelings congeal into a big undifferentiated lump.

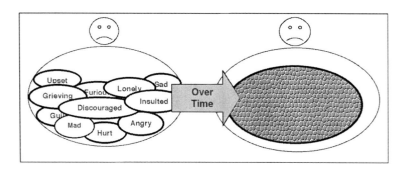

Eventually, this mass pollutes the entire interior space.

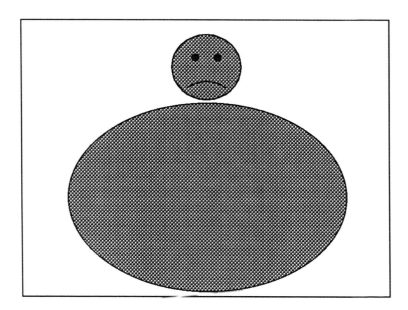

Some general average of these feelings, as well as a person's young training will cause him to let off stream in a recurring way, such that he sees himself—and others see him—as a label.

"I'm generally sad."

"He's an angry person."

"She's always depressed."

In fact, depression can be caused by a heavy blob of undifferentiated, unexpressed feeling, summarized as sad, tired, hopeless, or resigned. (Of course, *chemical* depression is a problem with neurotransmission delivery, and some people suffer from double depression, having both a chemical malfunction, *plus* a large lump of undifferentiated feeling.) We can melt the blob by learning to process our feelings.

This will be a critical skill for her to master, because one situation that can halt her progress is to be struck by a feeling that devastates her. For this reason, in her program she will be guided to handle difficult feelings in a healthy way.

She will learn to make a container [Agazarian, Systems-Centered® Training]xxxiv for her feelings so that she can experience the transformation that happens when feelings are processed. This allows one's inner landscape to calm..

Think of the difference between a meat press and a bowl—that's the difference between suppressing a feeling and creating a container for it. When we learn to contain feelings, we create interior space for it, letting it have the room it needs. This action allows feelings to release their encoded messages.

With practice, we get good at this and discover feelings as sources of wisdom and energy. Feelings are fluid. When they aren't blocked, they naturally flow into the next experience.

Your job is to encourage her to use her process. Most of all, don't say or do things that pilot her back into suppressing her feelings or experience.

Don't Say:

- You shouldn't feel that way.
- Calm down.
- Don't be so emotional.
- Eat this. You'll feel better.
- Let me kiss it away.
- You're being irrational.
- You're overreacting.
- You're too sensitive.
- You've always been this way.

Do:

- Support her as she practices the skills of healthy processing.
- Learn to listen in a way that enhances her discovery process. Next chapter, please.

27

The Stress Digester

Two communication skills are superb at helping others make room inside themselves for feelings: compassionate listening, xxxv xxxvi and functional subgrouping xxxvii [SCT®] xxxviii, xxxix [*Kudos to the brilliant minds that gave us process-centered learning—Dr. Alfred North Whitehead, and systems-centered® learning—Dr. Yvonne Agazarian, both fountainheads for ever-spreading ripples of increased therapeutic efficacy. A brief history of therapeutic listening can be found in the Appendix under "References".*]

Using these skills for your family can make a remarkable difference in the very atmosphere of your home. Everyone will benefit, especially if they've all been raised to avoid feelings.

Remember how it looks when feelings are avoided.

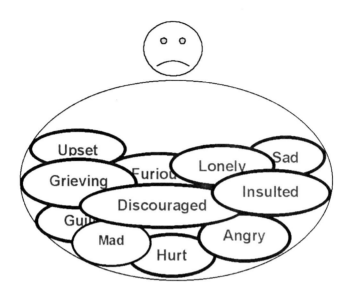

They can really build up. Notice the thick lines around each feeling. Those are defenses, boundaries so closed and thick that information and comfort can't get in or out.

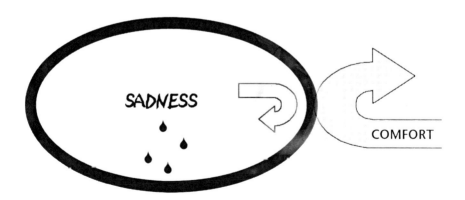

So what happens if the boundary is softened?

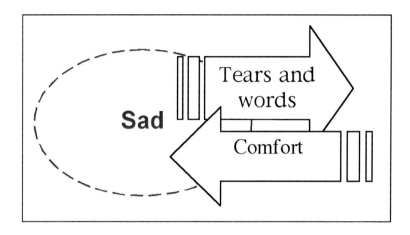

When the boundary relaxes, energy, information, and comfort can cross the membrane. (Just as we have the physics of mechanized motion or of quantum mechanics, we also now understand the physics of emotional health and relationships, drawing from the work of Yvonne Agazarian [Agazarian, 1997][xl].)

Naturally, our boundaries tighten when we are challenged, competed with, or met with criticism. They can relax when we are met with compassion.

Compassionate listening involves three parts:
- Creating an accepting space inside ourselves
- Listening to both words and expression
- Communicating accurate listening with compassion

Create an Accepting Internal Space

Calm yourself. Find the place inside where you are open and receptive to your loved one. Practice the discipline of containing your own feelings, so that you can be truly accepting of her process.

Listen to Both Words and Expression

Listen both to what she says and how she says it. What's the difference between the following examples?

Example 1. "I'm a little sad," she says, with a slight droop to her shoulders as she arranges flowers.

Example 2. "I'm a little sad," she says, sitting on the couch as she dabs the corner of her eye with a tissue.

Example 3. "I'm a little sad," she gasps, flinging herself across the bed and sobbing into her pillow.

Communicate Accurate Listening with Compassion

In Example 1, she's functioning and her body language is congruent with some sadness. If she uses busyness to avoid feeling, flower-arranging could be a sign that she's not letting herself really dip into what's going on. She might be holding back from being any more than just a little sad.

In this case, reflect the words, and make an offer. "I can see you're sad. Want to sit down and have some tea?" (*Having tea* is womanspeak for talking about real things, even if you end up drinking coffee.)

Example 2 is congruent. Her manner of expression, her words, and her actions all fit. She's already allowing herself to know what's going on. This is the easiest situation for you, because she isn't resisting herself. In this case, sit down and acknowledge her feelings. "You feel sad?"

People sometimes want to get fancy and embellish this, but actually, just a simple repeating of the main feeling is very powerful and signals acceptance.

In Example 3, everything but her words indicates a lot more than a little bit of sadness. Us stoic people tend to understate our feelings. We are making a bid for acceptance and comfort without taking too much risk at a vulnerable time. If you listen only to the words, you'll miss the mark.

In this case, sit down on the bed and reflect the behavior. "You are really, really sad."

Accurate listening means taking in the whole picture and reflecting that, including the feelings, the level of intensity, and the body language. Your tone of compassion, eye contact, and care are also a part of your message. Again, it doesn't have to be fancy. Simple words and simple comments invite her to continue.

And that's the point—for her to explore what's going on inside herself. You can tell you are doing a good job if her exploration advances. When she reacts to your listening with increased tears, a stream of words, or progression into other feelings like anger or grief, you are doing a good job. If she reacts by clamming up and turning away, you've missed somehow.

Think back to your tone and your words and discover if a criticism or judgment crept in. If you got uncomfortable with her intensity of feeling, did you say something to stop her.

That's okay. Just learn from it. Like any skill, accurate, compassionate listening takes a lot of practice. You'll have a learning curve and you'll get better at it.

Functional Subgrouping[xli]

This is a skill that changes one's whole attitude toward listening. (I have borrowed this, with permission, from systems-centered® training.) It automatically softens boundaries so that everyone has more access to information. It comes into its own in a group, such as a family, but it can be applied even to conflicts within yourself.

There are three parts to subgrouping, the join, the build, and passing the baton.

The Join

To join, you find something inside of you that is similar to what the other person just said.

"*I'm sad* that Mom can't come to our Thanksgiving dinner."

"*I'm sad too*, about Carl not coming."

In the above case, the feeling is shared and the reason is individual.

"I'm *sad that Mom can't come* to Thanksgiving."

"I *have feelings about Mom not coming too.* I experience them as this hot energy running up and down inside my chest."

Feelings about Mom are shared, and the bodily experience is individual.

The Build

With the build, you add information about your own feelings, experience, or exploration. In the examples below, the build will be in italics.

"I have feelings about Mom not coming too. *I experience them as this hot energy running up and down inside my chest.*"

"I have energy in my chest too, and *a heaviness. My eyes are prickling.*"

Passing the Baton

When you're through with your bit of exploration, indicate that you're ready to be joined by adding "anybody else?" Even if you're with just one other person, the intent is clear—that you're inviting the other person to find a way to join you, and that you have completed this portion of your exploration.

"I'm so excited about the new year. *I've got little arrows of energy darting all around inside me about the new class I'm taking.* Anybody else?"

"My energy is lively too. *I feel like dancing.* Anybody else?"

"I join you in having lively energy. *It's like lightning is racing through my arms and legs. I'm realizing my decision has freed my energy to do something new.* Anybody else?"

"I'm feeling good about my decision too. *I'm noticing that I feel like moving, like walking fast or running.* Anybody else?"

"I'm feeling a lot of energy in my arms, and it feels angry, like I want to punch the air. Anybody else?"

Silence.

As with compassionate listening, you can tell if a join and build are close enough to the spirit of the exploration by what happens after you pass the baton. If your build is close enough, others jump in and further the exploration. Together, you advance yourselves. If the build is too different, or if it's a "Yes, but," in disguise, the ball will drop.

In the above example, the introduction of angry energy stopped the process. The group was not ready for anger. However, if some of the others are on the edge of discovering their own anger, a new angry subgroup could form. It could proceed like this:

"I realize I have anger too. My insides are clenched and my hands want to shake something. Anybody else?"

"I'm angry. I want to stomp holes into the floor, anybody else?"

At this point, there are two subgroups, the angry subgroup and the excited subgroup. Each subgroup takes a turn to explore their emerging experience.

If you are with just one other person, it takes a little practice to find ways to authentically join the other person. Look for a side of the issue that you can genuinely join, explore it with her, and when that exploration is completed, you can bring up your other side of the same issue and explore that.

Communicating this way takes practice. We're more used to competing in conversation than cooperating. What begins to happen, though, is that boundaries open, more information is exchanged, and each person becomes capable of handling feelings that are more complex.

Choosing Your Method

After you've created a space for her to explore what's going on, should you listen or join? Let two things guide you. Your own level of comfort—choose the method that you are more comfortable with—and whether or not you are in her same boat.

If she's devastated that her best friend is moving and you never liked the woman anyway, it may be hard to find a way to join her feelings. Compassionate listening will be the way to go.

On the other hand, you both may be upset that the water treatment plant is being moved to your back yard. Functional subgrouping will work better since you have similar strong feelings.

You can also move back and forth between subgrouping and compassionate listening. Your goal is to assist her in moving through stress, and either process helps.

However, if you have genuine joins, not only will they help her move forward, your joins will reduce any sense of isolation. Plus, you'll learn something about yourself from your own joins and builds. An interesting benefit of functional subgrouping is that we begin to have access to our common sense, which may present us with a solution we would never have found otherwise.

Is Rescue a Remedy?

What about offering physical comfort, a hug or a snuggle?

Timing matters here. If tears are leaking silently from her eyes and you grab her and pull her into an embrace, she may get the message that you are uncomfortable with her feelings and want her to stop expressing them. She may then turn away from you when she's feeling vulnerable and look for someone else.

You're very good at fixing things. Should you fix the problem for her? What if she's been stepped on by her mean brother? Should you yell at him and take him down a peg? Will that help her?

The order in which you offer help makes a difference. Give her LOVE.

1. **Listen**
2. **Offer**
3. **Validate**
4. **Embrace**

Listen—You already know how to listen compassionately and to use subgrouping to advance both of you through a process of exploration.

Offer—Once you've listened and you are both complete around subgrouping, you can then offer other kinds of help. Be sure to wait until all exploration of feelings is complete before offering solutions. Always start your offer with an offer, "Would you like to hear a solution I thought of?"

Validate—Endorse her choice about her next move. If she wants to solve it herself rather than have you fix it, cheer her on. Let her know you believe in her.

Embrace—Now is the perfect time to offer her an embrace. She's processed her feelings, the two of you have developed a strategy, and now is a good time to ask if she'd like to be held. Your work is done and you might want to take some moments to relax together.

This order works in a variety of situations. At home, with plenty of time, each step can take as much time as necessary. Over tea in a Victorian tearoom, you can follow the same steps and give each as much time as you have. Even in a social situation like a family holiday dinner, the two of you can retreat to the porch and hit the highlights of each step. Just a lick and a promise can do a lot of good.

Your Tool Box

You have so much to offer when it comes to helping her reduce stress.
- Noticing clues that something's bothering her
- Making a space for her to talk
- Compassionate, accurate listening
- Functional subgrouping
- LOVE

28

The Breeder Reactor of Stress

Our families, God love them, can be a major source of stress. Events with the tribe offer great risk for relapse.

Families benefit enormously from the use of functional subgrouping, the skill you learned in the previous chapter, for it prevents scapegoating, increases common sense, and resolves conflict.

In the best of worlds, your whole family would go to a Systems-Centered® (SCT) therapist, workshop, or training, and learn the skill of functional subgrouping together. Failing that, you and your loved one can introduce functional subgrouping yourselves, by modeling it, especially when the family bully gets going.

A bully causes people to wall up their differences. His mean comments or strident opinions highjack air time. As you become easy with this skill, you can start a subgroup and offer silent members a safe way to join the quieter perspective. Done well, functional subgrouping creates an evolution of process that moves everyone to a more interesting and lively level. (This will be demonstrated in the next chapter.)

However, if you and your loved one are a subgroup of two, and the rest of the family unites to scapegoat one or both of you, it's okay to take the LOPE option.

Create a time-out. "Sami, could you help me find my gloves?" Go into an empty room and invite her to talk about what she's feeling.

Listen—as you know how to do

Offer—ask if she wants help handling the family or would it be better to leave the event

Plan a way to leave
Escape the family situation.

There's no dishonor in leaving a hostile situation. As Custer discovered, a timely retreat can make a big difference.

29

Family Fetes, Feasts and Fiestas

Curious?
Her family only wants what's best for her, right?
The one time she can safely eat sugar is
when her daughter bakes her first cookie, right?
Who is the most powerful person at family gatherings?

Any social event that has an abundance of food will be challenging for her, and most difficult of all will be family situations. No matter how evolved we are, when our family surrounds us, we slide down into old roles like on a greased rope.

If you grew up in this same family, you know this all too well. If you are her mate, then you've reaped the consequences of her family's beeswax one way or another.

In-laws are a challenge for her also. When she's around your family, she's an outsider to a certain extent, even if you've been married for years. Families don't always embrace spouses. In fact, there can be subtle currents of competition or rejection that hit her, but that you miss. Be on the look-out for these, and step in to support her.

Partnering her skillfully in your birth family can reap huge rewards in marital harmony and strengthen her recovery immeasurably. A wife who feels safe with you in the dire straits of hostile in-laws will be a wife who can risk the turbulent waters of recovery.

Here are some examples of comments that can steal her steel and threaten her eating plan.

"You've put on weight, haven't you?"

"He's gonna leave you if you don't lose weight."

"Your sister lost 20 pounds on that new 'Fist in Mouth' diet."

"That dress looks tight on you."

"You should never wear pants."

"That jacket looks so good on you. It hides your hips."

"Are you eating *again*?"

"Why did you bring your own food. Isn't mine good enough?"

"I guess you're too hoity-toity to eat ordinary sandwiches like the rest of us."

"I made this cake just for you."

"Have some brownies. I know they are your favorite."

"I stayed on my feet all day to fix this candy for you."

"You don't want these rolls, Mama? It's the best thing I cook."

"You have the same shape as Aunt Gert. She's built like a truck too."

"Even when you were a little girl, you had to be different."

"Just have one bite. One bite can't kill you."

"I read about this new diet and I thought of you. It sounds like a good one."

"I got these pills that help people lose ten pounds a week. I got enough for you too."

From her brother-in-law, sotto voce, standing too close, "Hey, sugar, you've lost some weight. And you're looking good. *Real* good."

How You Can Help

Reach for her hand. With one simple gesture you can both indicate solidarity and re-connect her to the reality that exists outside this family cobweb. In an instant, she is reassured that she is not alone and is reminded that she has another life beyond these walls.

Create a time-out. "Honey, could you help me with something?" Give her a way to leave the situation. As she gets close to you, take her arm and go into another room or take a short walk. Offer an ear and let her talk about her reaction to the way she's being treated. Give LOVE (Listen, Offer, Validate, Embrace).

LOPE is always an option (Listen, Offer, Plan, Escape). If she needs to leave to keep from being traumatized or victimized, that's okay. Her recovery is more important than this family occasion.

Enter her subgroup. Join her side of the situation by making a comment that publicly aligns you with her, and at the end, add "Anybody else?" This invites others to stand with the two of you. As explained in Chapter 28, the point of this is not to create factions, but to make differences acceptable.

If you are willing, intercede with protective or instructive comments. In the next section are sample dialogues that demonstrate responses you could make. You do not have to memorize them. Just read them and get a feel for the various directions support can go. After the examples, I'll explain the principles behind the responses.

Difficult or hurtful remarks can be sorted into categories. These are:

- Criticism, complaints, or comparisons
- Intrusive, mean, or sexual comments
- Food pushing, manipulation, or power plays
- Pure ignorance
- Innocent or well-meaning comments or gifts

Criticism, Complaints, or Comparisons

In each instance, remarks are said in a critical tone and initially addressed to your loved one. Your supportive responses are in bold type.

Example 1. "That dress looks tight on you." Or, "You should never wear pants."
"Please stop making any comments about her appearance.
"I didn't mean anything by it."
"Regardless, stop please."

Example 2. "You have the same dumpy shape as my mother."
"She has the same kindness, that's for sure. But stop comparing her to other people, Mom. Keep those thoughts to yourself.
"Can't I say what I want to in my own house?"

"You can, but we can also go to a place where we don't have to hear words that hurt."

"Oh, is she *sensitive*?"

"She's too kind to return your rudeness with more rudeness, but neither one of us is willing to be put down."

Example 3. "Your sister lost 20 pounds on that new 'Fist in Mouth' diet."

"Good for her. It couldn't have been easy. We all have a malfunctioning appetite switch."

Example 4. "Are you eating *again*?"

"Does that bother you?"

"Well, I cooked all day, and now she won't want what I'm fixing."

"All the rest of us definitely want what you're fixing. She is taking care of herself. If you are interested, we'll explain it sometime."

Example 5. "You aren't going to eat pasta like we are? Even when you were a little girl, you had to be different."

"Ouch."

"What?"

"That wasn't even directed at me and I felt bad immediately."

"What'd I say?"

"You made her wrong for taking care of herself."

"Now you're going to start on me."*

"Okay, I'm pulling out of this conversation, but she and I are going for a walk. Meanwhile, please stop criticizing us. As much as we love you and want to be here, we're both leaving if this keeps up."

"Is that a threat?"

"It's a boundary. See you in a bit."

Criticisms and comparisons can render the target speechless. They can slam into a person so hard that she can't think how to take care of herself. Even though it's the comment—rather than anything about her—that is in the wrong, she can feel shamed, as if she has to defend herself.

Swift intervention on your part can accomplish a lot. First, it gives her some room to recover from the hostility embedded in the comment. Second, it serves notice that you will not allow her to be made a scapegoat by the family. Third, you demonstrate that you will bring the truth into the open even if the criticizer is concealing his motive for saying hurtful things.

In examples 1 and 2, you immediately set a boundary. (It's easier to say you than "the responder" or "her husband, sister, or brother.")

Notice, in neither case did you engage with the criticism. Sometimes people are just looking for a fight. For some people, a fight feels like intimacy and engagement.

In example 2, when the first attack failed, the mother switched to another angle of attack. Each of these was met with a boundary.

Example 3 demonstrates another type of response that can work if you can feel light-hearted in delivering it. It's a deliberate misreading of the criticism, vectoring the conversation toward a positive slant. This can muddle the criticizer just enough to successfully change the subject.

Example 4 demonstrates yet another technique: exploring the person's motive in making the comment. If a person's concern can be revealed, it may be possible to meet it, which can then remove their impetus for retaliation.

Example 5 is a particularly powerful type of support. It legitimizes the target's hurt feelings and names the potshot directed at her.

Sometimes a bully has everyone in the family so cowed that no one rises to the defense of the target, partly from being shocked and rendered speechless, partly from a long-standing pattern of caving under intimidation. Then the bully gets away with abuse one more time. Verbalizing the consequence of the hit, "Ouch," can push others out of shock and rally the family's courage.

Notice in this example, the bully did a bait and switch, first acting innocent as if she hadn't done anything, and then acting victimized when she was called on it. (The remark with the asterisk.)

When someone pulls a bait and switch, that's your notice that conversation is not going to work. This person is sliding around the abuse triangle, pretending to be victimized when she herself has been the abuser. (The three points on the abuse triangle are victim, abuser, caretaker.)

At this point you cleverly refused any more engagement, created a boundary through a time-out, and set a stronger boundary should the unacceptable behavior continue.

Intrusive, mean, or sexual comments

Intrusive, mean, or sexual remarks are all a form of attack. Like the comments in the above section, they can cause a person to freeze and to be unable to access her usual ability to protect herself.

These may also, like the previous examples, be critical or introduce a comparison. When two forms of attack are hurled at someone—such as both a mean comment and a comparison, if you can, set the boundary for the most hurtful one. The lesser aspect then automatically gets fenced out by the boundary.

Comments about size, weight, appearance, and food choices are intrusive. Even a compliment can sometimes embed a sly needle. Don't let these pass. Make it clear that these comments are not okay.

Example 6. "You have the same shape as Aunt Gert. She's built like a hydrant too."
"Why would you say something like that to her, Dad? Please stop. That can only hurt.
"I'm just telling the truth."
"Like I'd be telling the truth if I said you started drinking too early today and it's already affecting your judgment?"
"I can do what I want. This is my house."
"Okay, you stick to your business and we'll stick to ours."
"I still say she's built like a hydrant."
"Enough. We're leaving."

Example 7. "You've put on weight, haven't you?"
"Whoa, Mom, not okay."
"I've got eyes, haven't I?"

"Mom, every time we come, you comment about my wife's weight. This has to stop. I won't stand for her to be treated unkindly by my family."

"I knew she'd steal you away from us."

"Sounds like you think you're in competition with each other."**

"What?"

"You don't have to compete. I love you and I love her."

"I love you too, Son."

"Are you willing to stop making comments about her weight?"

"You know, that's the first thing your dad's mom always said to me. I guess I was just passing it on."

"Did it hurt you when Granny said that?"

"Of course it did. I didn't even want to visit them for the longest time."

"Uh-huh. Same goes."

"I apologize, Tania. I wasn't thinking. I'll make an effort to not do it again, and if I do, make a big face at me to get my attention."

"Good going, Mom. Give me a hug."

Example 8. "He's gonna leave you if you don't lose weight."

"Mom-in-law, look over here. That's not going to happen. You don't need to fear for her."

"Honestly, Ed, aren't you ashamed to be seen with her?"

"You mean like when she's leading the fund drive for orphaned kids, or singing in the choir, or standing out in subzero weather to make sure Jason gets safely on the bus?"

"How about when you go to dances at the officer's club?"

"You mean when I waltz my wife across the floor and she's the most graceful one there?"

"I don't see how it doesn't bother you."

"My wife and your daughter is so much more than skin deep. And I'm surprised you're criticizing her, because in fact she has lost weight. But whether she has or not, what's important to me is what a wonderful person she is. And that she's such a good mother. I'm proud of her. Anybody else?"

Example 9. "That jacket looks so good on you. It hides your hips."

"Whoa, Bettina, not worthy of ya."
"What?"
"Putting poison in the apple."
"What are you talking about?"
"Okay. End of discussion. No comments about my sister's body. Period. Zip. Nadda."

Example 10. From her brother-in-law, sotto voce, standing too close, "Hey, sugar, you've lost some weight. And you're looking good. *Real* good."
Moving to block him from getting closer to her, "Stop. Now and always."
"Hey, I didn't mean nothing."
"No more. Never talk to my wife like that again. Never."
"All right. All right. I didn't know you were so touchy."
"Never."

In example 6, it was irresistible to engage in argument. Sometimes we just won't be able to help it when a criticism is so blatantly cruel. If the person persists and is totally unwilling to respect the boundary that has been set, then removing yourself from the situation is the best option.

In example 7, you set two boundaries immediately, in between, calling attention to a previous boundary violation that was now being repeated. In the next comment, you brilliantly go to the heart of the problem (double asterisk). This changes the tide of the conversation and brings a completely unexpected outcome.

A conversion is possible if we can relax enough to perceive what is behind an attack and then turn the dialogue toward what is really at stake for the attacker. Not everyone will be willing to look at themselves or be able to trace where their hurtful behavior originates, but this dialogue introduces the idea of rewarding approximations of the desired behavior. Each time Mom opened, her son drew closer to her, which is what Mom wanted all along.

A person who hasn't practiced healthy dialogue may make a lot of mistakes as they are learning, just as we all do when we learn a new skill. So, rather than expecting perfection, support their learning by responding warmly when they are nudging toward the healthier direction.

Example 8 is a similar effort. You respond with a testing comment. If what's going on with Mom is that she's fearful for her daughter, the response lays that to rest.

It turns out Mom is just mean. Further rebuttal doesn't make any difference to her. She keeps on attacking. It's time for a boundary or creating a subgroup and that's what you do, creating a 'proud of her' subgroup and inviting alignment from other family members.

Example 9 blows the whistle and sets a boundary.

Example 10 protects her sexually. Since many women are fearful of losing weight precisely because of such unwelcome sexual attention, it is very important that you intervene strongly and decisively. Forget diplomacy, forget about trying to preserve peace in the family.

Sexual predators get power from silence so don't let it pass, don't excuse it. Set a non-negotiable boundary and protect her. You will be such a hero.

Remember this about bullies. They attack because they feel weak. If you stand up strongly to a bully, they will back down. If you also give the rest of the family a way to join you in protecting your loved one, the bully will back down even faster.

(Don't expect a healthy or gracious retreat from them. They'll go out with a potshot or by pretending to be victimized. Let that go. Don't try to enlighten them. With a bully who is making no effort toward self-improvement, the goal is to detach and disengage. Let them have the empty victory of the last word.)

Food Pushing, Manipulation, or Power plays

Sometimes food pushing is benign or because the cook's identity is wrapped up in her product. Sometimes it's a disguised effort to control the other person. If you can sense which motive is at work, it can guide your response—whether to set a boundary or to make an attempt to educate or soothe the pusher.

Example 11. "Just have one bite. One bite can't kill you."

"Mother, are you thinking you are helping Sarie?"

"I made this scrumptious dessert and she's not even going to try it."

"It sounds like you might like some appreciation."

"Well, yes. I put a lot of effort into these holidays."

"I know you do. I'm loving this meal. I know how hard you work to make it nice. Can my appreciation make up for Sarie not having any dessert?"

"I still don't understand why she can't have at least a small serving."

"I'll be happy to explain it if you like."

"Okay, after dinner you tell me about it."

Example 12. "Why did you bring your own food. Isn't mine good enough?" (Passive-aggressive, determined-to-be-victimized tone.)

"Your food is very good, Aunt Martyr. It's just that we're both eating differently now and we didn't want to put you out."

"So I guess you're saying my food isn't healthy."

"Is that what you are hearing?"

"Kids," raising her voice, "your cousins don't want to eat the good dinner I slaved over. I knew when Bryan married her, she'd be picky."

"Oops, you crossed the line, Aunt Martyr. It's not okay with me for you to criticize my wife, or to make her at fault when all we're doing is finding a way to share this holiday with you while still taking care of ourselves. I'm sorry you're taking this personally when it isn't about you. And it's too bad you can't see that our main focus is to be here with you."

"You do run on, Bryan, I don't know what all you're talking about."

"I'm saying, Aunt Martyr, please don't make a big deal out of what we're choosing to eat, and do not criticize my wife."

"Well, all right, then. You always had to have your way."

"What can we do to help get things ready?"

Example 13. "Why did you bring your own food. Isn't mine good enough?" (Mean, aggressive, looking-for-a-fight tone.)

"You're a great cook, Aunt Pugnacious. We've both been eating differently lately and we didn't want to put you out."

"You could have told me. I made all this extra food that will go to waste."

"Actually, Beth called a couple of times to let you know in advance."

"Well, I've been busy. I have a life too, you know. I can't sit around waiting for the phone to ring."

"Of course you can't. How can we help you get ready?"

"Did you think I wouldn't have things ready?"

"Thanks for doing so much. We'll be with our cousins. Call if you need help."

"Do I look weak to you?"

Example 14. "I guess you're too hoity-toity to eat ordinary sandwiches like the rest of us."

"That's one possibility."

"You're being sarcastic."

"I suppose I am. I get tired of you labeling my sister when she's got the courage to be changing her life.

Example 15. "I made this cake just for your birthday." Or "Have some brownies, I know they are your favorite."

"Aunt Needy, thank you so much. That was very generous. I just want to say once again that Talia is on a food plan that prevents diabetes. The best birthday present you could give her would be to cut up some of those apples and throw in some little slices of cheese."

"What about the candles?"

"Put one in a square of cheese."

"What am I going to do with this cake?"

"How about I come by tomorrow and take it to the office with me. I can assure you it will be enjoyed."

"What if you can't make it, then what will I do?"

Example 16. "I stayed on my feet all day to fix this candy for her."

"Mama, look at me for a second. Jayla isn't eating sugar. We talked about this last time. What's making it hard for you to remember this?"

"It's what we've always done."

"Are you having a hard time thinking how else to give to us?"

"That's part of it."

"It would be a gift to us just to sit down with you and talk."

"But I like to do things before you come. I plan and cook and think about you while you're traveling here."

"I get it Mama. It makes the visit longer and it brings us here in your thoughts as you're cooking."

"That's right."

"Well how about cooking turkey? On our new plan, we eat a lot of turkey. You could cook turkey for us and that would be a real gift."

"But it's not Thanksgiving."

"Would it be okay with you if we made a new tradition?"

"I suppose we could do that."

"You could enjoy cooking the turkey ahead of time and we'd get to eat home-cooked food that we really need."

"With dressing and cranberry sauce."

"Oh, I'm glad you mentioned that. Let's start a new tradition there too. We aren't eating bread and cranberry sauce has sugar in it."

"No dressing?"

"What if you made a dressing out of brown rice?"

"And I could add dried apricots to it, and raisins."

"Mama, if I gave you a list of what we eat and what we don't eat, would you be willing to figure out how to make a new kind of dressing."

"Of course I would. I'd enjoy that."

"Thanks a lot, Mama. It's not easy to change a long tradition, but this would be great for us."

"And we could have turkey sandwiches and turkey casserole with potato chips, and …"

"Mama, remember, no bread."

"Oh, right. I'll have to do some thinking about this."

"Mama, you're the greatest. I have to kiss your cheek."

"Go on," she waves her hand at you while offering her cheek and a touching smile.

In example 11, your probing comment exposes that Mother feels put upon and unappreciated. Your instant appreciation soothes her enough to be able to take in information about this different way of eating.

Aunt Martyr, in example 12, is determined to be victimized. Nothing you can do but set a boundary, put some teeth in it, and change the subject.

Aunt Pugnacious, example 13, is looking for a fight. She can twist any generosity on your part into an insult and she will always have the last word. You get a Nobel prize for not decking her. You might as well take care of yourselves, because nothing will make her happy anyway. Oh, and consider reducing your contacts with her.

Example 14 demonstrates non-resistance. You won't be any fun to a person seeking a power struggle so she will soon move onto more interesting game.

In example 15, Aunt Needy wields the power of the insistently helpless person. Her indirect anger has you tap-dancing while she claps the rhythm. Here, you are offering solutions to the faux problems she is presenting. If she continues to hold you in thrall with endless problems, end the dialogue with a choice and a departure: "Aunt Needy, I can pick up the cake tomorrow or you can find someone else who will enjoy it. I'm going to join the others now. Let me know what you decide."

It is really tempting to tell her just what she can do with her precious cake, but it doesn't actually work to feed food in from the bottom of the anatomy. If you start to feel angry, requiring severe self-discipline to keep from lashing out, know that you are now carrying the anger that she is unable to express. This is her feeling, not yours. Get out of the situation immediately. It is not necessary to be polite when you are being manipulated.

Example 16 is food pushing from the most innocent of motives: a desire to give, to connect, and to express love. Through truly superb listening, you get to the heart of the matter and offer a compromise that blesses both sides, giving everyone involved what they most need.

Pure Ignorance

Remember you are blazing a trail. Lots of people have never heard of food addiction or the appetite switch. When a person is simply uninformed, with no meanness or hidden agenda, offering information can be helpful to everyone.

Example 17. "Are you eating again?" she says with a questioning tone, no meanness.

"Sis, we're on a new eating program. We both have realized we have a stuck appetite switch and we're fixing it. We eat more often, and then we end up eating less."

"Never heard of such a thing."

"It's working well for us. But it's still hard when people don't understand, and when they put a spotlight on us for eating differently."

"I'm sorry. I didn't know."

"Of course you didn't. But what would help is if you just let us take care of ourselves and not make a big deal of it."

"Well, I have problems with my appetite too now that I think about it. So I'm interested in what you're doing. Maybe it would help me too."

"Hey, join us. The more we support each other, the easier it is."

Example 18. "I thought she liked bread?"

"It turns out that bread makes her eat more than she wants to. So the way she can have peace around eating is to have no bread at all."

"No bread at all?"

"None."

"And what do you do? You love bread."

"I do, and so I eat my bread when I'm not with her."

"Is she too weak to see you eat it?"

"It's not weakness, Sis, it's a chemical reaction. Just seeing food can trigger her to eat too much, especially if she's in a place where she's vulnerable. At home she lets down her defenses, so if I eat bread in front of her there, she starts wanting it."

"What about sandwiches? You love sandwiches."

"That's true. So I have a sandwich every day at work. I can eat as many sandwiches as I want, away from home."

"You sure are sacrificing a lot for her."

Laughing. "You're not trying to get me to resent her, are you? Or drive a little split between us?"

"Gorgio, what a thing to say." Pause. "You're giving me a look. Okay, maybe a little. She's not one of us, and not eating bread is a big deal in our family."

"Sis, doesn't it strike you as odd that eating or not eating a mere food should be a big deal?"

"Okay, big brother. I'll think about this. You're a good husband. I'm proud of you."

"Thanks, I'm proud of you too, for being honest and for talking this out with me. So, please, help me stand up for her if Mama puts pressure on her to eat the bread at dinner."

"You bet, big guy. Should be entertaining."

Example 19. "These pills guarantee you'll lose ten pounds a week. Here, I got them for you."

"Hold on there, Jasmine. What are you giving to my wife?"

"I'm giving *my sister* something to help her with her weight."

"Let me look at those things."

"Can't Lotus speak for herself?"

"She did. Did you hear her?"

"What are you talking about?"

"When you first brought it up, she said clearly she wasn't interested in taking them."

"I thought she didn't understand how good they are."

"She doesn't want to take them."

"Why are you butting in?"

"Because I want to support her. Those kinds of pills are the ones that cause a rebound of eating. Sooner or later, you either have to take more or go off them. Either way, it's not good for her."

"Well, if the two of you are going to gang up on me, I guess I'll just keep these for myself. You'll be sorry when you see how thin I get."

"I'll be sorry if they aren't good for you either."

Example 20. "Just have one bite. One bite can't kill you."
"Aunt Generous, you mean well, but one bite of sugar could actually kill her, eventually."
"You don't mean that."
"I do. I'm going to tell you something private, just for you to know. Shasta and I agreed before we got here that I would explain it. For Shasta, even a small amount of sugar triggers her appetite, and then no amount of will power can overcome her desire to eat."
"I had no idea."
"She's being very polite and keeps saying no, but I thought if you understood why she's declining your dessert, you might stop tempting her with it."
"Darling, I meant you no harm. What would you like instead?"

In example 17, you stick up for her while offering information. It opens a door for your sister to address her own appetite switch and to join you in eating differently.

In example 18, your sister gets a little competitive with your wife and tries to pull you into feeling sorry for yourself. You counter masterfully using logic and humor to call her on her ploy. Then you point out a family quirk that would have made a scapegoat of your wife, widening your sister's perception. This leads to a leavening for all and a plan for extended support for your wife.

Example 19 is a combination of good solid support and information, and example 20 is what's possible with a truly well-meaning person who just doesn't know about the appetite switch or food addiction. Notice that you and Shasta planned ahead of time what private information you would reveal so that you are modeling appropriate boundaries around privacy with Aunt Generous and conveying the privilege you are bestowing on her by taking her into your confidence.

Innocent or well-meaning comments or gifts

Not surprisingly, food presented with love and generosity is the hardest to deal with. Our boundaries close when arrows fly, but for roses we open. You can be of tremendous help here, because this could be the one comment that could get past her commitment to abstinence.

Example 21. "You don't want these rolls, Mama? It's the best thing I cook."

"Honey, you may not realize that your mother is doing something great for herself. She's treating her appetite disorder, and as much as she wants to try what you've made, if she had even one bite, she could have a real hard time getting back to her eating plan. I know you don't wish that for her."

"But Daddy, I wanted to show off my baking, plus, my rolls are the best part of the meal."

"Sweetheart, I'll enjoy your rolls. And because she loves you, she might have eaten one and then gotten off her plan. The best thing about this meal is that we're all together here in your first apartment."

"Do you really not want a roll, Mama?"

Your wife answers, "I do, honey, that's why your dad is helping me. I would eat it and then I might not be able to stop eating them. I'm addicted to bread of all kinds."

"I never heard of that."

"Your mom just can't eat bread anymore. She wants to be as healthy as possible. Would you join me in supporting her?"

"Of course, Daddy. I want you healthy, Mama."

* * *

Example 22. "Why did you bring your own food. Isn't mine good enough?" (Hurt tone.)

"It's too good, Aunt Tender. We're both eating differently now and we knew we'd be too tempted by your good cooking if we didn't bring something on our plan."

"I can cook whatever you can eat. Tell me about your plan and next time my menu will be what you can eat. I'm sure it would be good for me too."

"You're the best, Aunt Tender."

Example 23. "I read about this new diet and I thought of your wife. It sounds like a good one. I brought a copy for you to give to her."

"You mean well, Amrita , but Ila and I are both looking at food differently these days."

"What do you mean?"

"She has been on lots of diets and every time they haven't worked. Now we realize our old way of eating isn't good for us at our age. Ila has switched from dieting to eating in a different way, and I support her."

"Well, I'll just tell her about it. Then she can try it when she gets done with the diet she's on now."

"Amrita, do you want to support what's good for her?"

"But of course."

"Then don't tell her about any diet. Instead, you might ask her to talk about how she has been feeling lately. And we plan to continue eating this way from now on."

Principles for Responding

- If it's an attack, set a boundary. If it isn't respected, make it stronger.
- If the attack is sexual in nature, protect her immediately.
- If the person is mean, manipulative, drunk, or acting out some kind of power play, disengage as soon as possible. Techniques for disengagement include:
  - ○ Distraction: Changing the subject or offering to help.
  - ○ Humor: Diverting attention or changing the intensity.
  - ○ Non-resistance: Moving in the same direction as the punch.
  - ○ Offering a choice, letting them be in charge of when they give you the answer, and then leaving the room or conversation.
  - ○ Leaving the situation either permanently or temporarily.
- If you perceive that the comment is coming from an unmet need and you value the relationship enough to stretch yourself, you can help the person explore the need and, if you feel comfortable, meet the need in some way. In this case, you'll need your best listening skills. (Chapter 27.)

- If this person has a record of being able to work things out, you may be able to:
  - ○ Call them on their behavior.
  - ○ Negotiate solutions.
  - ○ Offer information or education
- If this is a truly well-meaning person, explore together how everyone's needs can be met.

The more willing you are to stick up for her, the stronger she'll get in following her recovery program. And your efforts will strengthen your mutual relationship as well. Many wives, sisters, mothers, and daughters would be overwhelmed with gratitude with this kind of solid support.

Supporting her recovery in a family situation wins you an Oscar for "Best Husband/Sister/Partner/Mother/Father/Brother/Daughter or Son."

30
The Sabotaging Family

Alie had been abstinent for almost two years. She had worked her program assiduously through that time and now looked forward to a visit from her family. Her mom and dad, her brother and his wife, their three sons—they were all converging for a reunion. She was a wonderful aunt, great with kids, and she adored her nephews and they loved her.

Her mom was a bit of a food pusher, but she was starting to understand food addiction. Before she came, she even asked Alie to remind her what foods she could eat. Alie was pleased that her mother finally wanted to support her.

The reunion started well. Everyone was glad to be together. They had warm, relaxed conversations and plenty of laughter.

Then her dad asked Alie to pick up the tickets he'd ordered for the ball game. The highlight of the visit was to go the new baseball stadium and watch a major league game, her dad's treat. Alie picked up the tickets, and then counted them. There were seven. She said to the vendor. "We're missing a ticket."

She checked her computer. "No, Ma'am, only seven tickets were ordered."

Alie thought for a few seconds. She was sure they didn't mean to leave the youngest son at home alone. She said, "I'm sure it's a mistake. I'll buy another ticket."

"No more tickets, Ma'am. We're sold out."

Alie couldn't imagine what her dad's plan was. She went home and found everyone sitting around the living room. "Dad, they only had seven tickets. Does someone not want to go?"

Her dad put down the paper. He had a strange look on his face. She suddenly knew. He'd forgotten her.

"You wouldn't want to go anyway, would you?" He said belligerently.

"To be there the first time my nephews go to a real ballpark? To watch my nephews see their first major league game? Not to mention that I like baseball? Yes, I want to go."

He said crossly, "Well, why didn't you buy another ticket?"

She was speechless. How was she in the wrong? Her mother, brother, and sister-in-law were all watching, and they said nothing.

She finally said, "They're sold out."

He got up blustering. "Well I'll find another ticket."

But he couldn't. They really were sold out.

Her dad's way of handling this sad outcome was to say, "You wouldn't have been able to sit with us anyway." And the ensuing silence of the rest of the family made them complicit.

I wondered, when I heard this story later, why they didn't insist she go with them anyway. There are always scalpers outside the gate. If I'd been the parent that miscounted and left out my daughter, I'd pay the inflated price to make sure she was included. If I found a ticket, we'd all take turns sitting in the single seat away from the others. And if no ticket were to be had, I'd take the consequence myself.

This is a good example of a child being treated as the Cinderella of the family. To make such a blatant error and then not to go to any length to fix it, making her wrong in the process, is the kind of thing that wounds very deeply.

Alie's abstinence began to crumble almost immediately. She tried to enjoy the rest of the reunion, but she was so hurt, it colored the remainder of the visit. It took her a long time to find her anger, but by then, her abstinence was gone. This was a wound that made recovery pale in significance.

You love an overeater. Her family has so much power. If you find yourself in a situation with her that resembles Alie's treatment, stick up for her. The entire course of the reunion would have been changed if someone else had spoken. If her brother had said, "Dad, let's find a solution. Let's go early. There's bound to be a scalper. I'll pitch in to pay for it."

Or her mother had said, "George, we can't leave her out. Don't you know somebody who knows somebody?"

Or her dad had said, "You know what? It's my mistake. Alie, you go with us. If we can't find a ticket, you take mine. I'll go to Mulligan's and watch it from there."

It's easy to say that it's up to Alie to protect her abstinence. That's true. But it's also true that we are all vulnerable to certain blows and can be felled by them. When the bottom drops out, it's hard to remember that satiety chemicals matter.

Your intervention is crucial in these situations. Muster your strength and common sense and either support her or help her to leave the room so she can regroup.

Some families are so sick that your recovering overeater will never be safe with them, no matter how far along she is in her recovery. Help her keep perspective if she drifts into a fantasy that her family will magically be kinder now that she has been in recovery.

Her family isn't mean because she eats. Initially, she probably ate because her family was mean. They have the power to trigger her again. When this is the case, the answer is to stay away.

(This is a very important and serious decision—to stay away in order to protect abstinence. All overeaters have occasional slips—it's just part of the disorder. However, a true relapse is another beast. After a person has had an extended period of good abstinence, a relapse can last for years. It's shockingly easy to lose an established abstinence, and unbelievably difficult to re-achieve that same level of abstinence—especially when the cause of the relapse is severe wounding from someone she loves.)

Recovery means life. Protecting life is the priority.

31

Handling Your Anger

This chapter is just for you. It's your opportunity to release your anger for the trouble her appetite disorder has caused you.

Here is where you get to say whatever you think about this aggravating disorder even if it's not politically correct. You don't have to be careful with words. You don't even have to keep your voice down if you do this work when no one is home or when you're with a buddy in the same boat.

Here are a few boundaries for your and her protection. Say and feel whatever you like, but don't express it in this way to her. Give yourself the freedom to have your whole experience, and then decide later what part you will share.

In a previous chapter, you learned about containing feelings rather than suppressing them. Another discipline regarding feelings is to contain them rather than act them out. To act out a feeling includes lashing out, setting someone up, venting rage without restraint, making a passive aggressive comment, and being sarcastic or critical.

I encourage you to express your feelings fully about the issues aroused by her disorder, either to a friend, therapist, mentor, or pastor, without acting them out on her.

Are you angry? I don't blame you. I'm angry too.

How many times have you endured the cabbage soup diet or bought special foods or tried to follow rules set up by her latest diet fad? How many diet programs have you funded?

The first times you were so supportive of her. You put up with grapefruit three times a day or sat alone at the table while she drank her special shake and left the kitchen. You shopped and cleaned up. You made peanut butter sandwiches for the kids. You took her shopping for new clothes. You blotted her tears.

Of course you're burned out on supporting her through one more complicated program. Haven't all the others led to a dubious outcome? Hasn't she failed time and time again?

Feel free to list all the irritating, frustrating, aggravating adjustments you've made because of her appetite disorder. Notice the sensations in your body. Make room for them. Express them.

If you're a wordsmith, write down all the ways you've tried to help her and the metaphors that express your feelings. If you're a geek, make a spreadsheet. If you're a gardener, channel your energy into attacking weeds. If you're an artist, draw a scene, a montage, or make a mosaic. If you're a sports fan, imagine that the opposing team is the appetite disorder.

Get it out somehow, in words, gestures, shouts, pictures, or heated conversation with a friend. Give yourself all the time you need.

Your anger is appropriate. I join you in it. I'm angry. I feel like taking the diet industry in my hands and shaking it. I want to say to them, "You've made billions off the backs of women who trusted you. You've put ingredients in your diet foods that made them gain weight and stay addicted to food. You've made them the scapegoat, as if they are weak for not staying on your diet, when the diet itself set them up to relapse." I want to say to a few (but not all) medical folks, "You blamed your patient when it became clear that a universally-prescribed remedy wasn't effective without careful preparation and informed, sustained support," and to the culture at large, "I'm angry at the strange blindness that causes you to heap so much blame on heavy people, when they are clearly already suffering."

And I notice the hot energy in my body, as if there is lightning in my hands and as I wave my arms, bolts of jagged light shoot from my fingers. Anybody else?

32

The Crucial Shift

For decades we've thought of obesity as being a consequence of overeating, thus we thought a diet would solve the problem. And as long as we continue to think that way, we'll perpetuate the problem.

The reality is, obesity is a consequence of chemically-forced feeding, suppressed metabolism, resistance to exercise, delayed or malfunctioning satiety chemicals, damaged leptin receptors, hypothalamic lesions, and a depletion of dopamine D-2 receptors.

It takes practice to think in a different way, to think of overeating as a consequence of chemicals that drive feeding. But making this shift in perception is crucial, because only by really grasping it, will we pay attention to the right problem.

I know it took me a long to time to get it. I had to undo an automatic thought that said eating was bad. I finally learned to use my eating behavior as a signpost as to what was going on with me chemically. Thinking this way pointed me toward fixing the errant chemical.

Are you willing to make room in your mind for this revolution of thought? Doing so will lead you to a very different and much more effective path than the dead-end of the diet mentality.

Diet Mentality

Restrictive
Depriving
White knuckles
Hunger
Being a "Good Girl"
The diet will come to an end.
After the diet is over, she can eat what she wants.

Chemical-balancing Mentality

Fix the appetite switch.

> Lower NPY, orexins, ghrelin, and addictive chemicals.
> Increase PYY, cholescystokinin, and serotonin.
> Counteract norepinephrine.
> Protect and nurture her satiety chemicals.

Eat in a way that meets those goals.

If appetite increases, look around to see what part of the program got dropped.

When stress increases, increase support and tryptophan.

Remember that this is a lifelong process and if she slips up or gets lax, she just returns to her program.

This is the shift she'll have to transit, and the challenge is for you to make the same shift. Do you have an automatic reflex when you see her eating? Do you have an instant reaction of disapproval or dismay?

It's understandable, but if she is following a program to heal her appetite disorder, use your mind to bring yourself into the new reality. Your mental shift can move from, "Oh, no, she's eating again," to, "Good, she's snacking to protect her satiety."

Protecting satiety—that's the name of the game. Protect those brain chemicals that stop overeating.

Any failure she has had in sustaining a diet is due to the fact that she has run into a wall of chemicals that bounced her back into the food. Neither of you can push through that wall, but, together, you can dismantle it. Just remember that her program must be sustained or the wall will grow back.

Do:

- Support her in continuing with her support group
- Find a way to occupy yourself if she needs to spend some time on the phone each day with her support buddy.
- Remember that in the long run, recovery is economical. A few hours each week of support yields a healthier, more available loved one.
- Remember: health is a cost saver. Illness is expensive.

Don't:

- Don't take it personally if she needs to run certain issues by her support group before she brings them to you.
- Don't get competitive with her support buddy or group. She needs all of you.

33

Getting What You Want

I want consistency around what she can eat and what I can share with her.

Part I:

✓ She can eat three meals and two snacks.

✓ All meals and snacks must include some protein.

✓ Snacks must not contain any sugar, flour, or wheat.

✓ No food or drink can contain NutraSweet, equal, or msg.

Quiz Question:

She slips. She's been abstinent from sugar, but she eats a cookie. Does this mean you can now offer her cookies? (See the answer at the end of Part II.)

Part II:

✓ Once she is abstinent, don't offer her any food from which she is abstinent.

By continuing to support her abstinence (thus refusing to enable her), you can have the consistency you want. [Answer: No. Once you know her list of not-safe foods, never offer them again, not even if she slips or relapses.]

(For a model of the effectiveness of not enabling, remember, if you are old enough, what happened with smokers when the United States made smoking inconvenient. Gradually, smoking was prohibited in more and more places—airplanes, public buildings, businesses, sports venues, restaurants, and even some bars—and more and more smokers quit.

The culture stopped enabling smokers [thus forcing them to experience withdrawal over and over] and many smokers became non-smokers.)

I want consistent limits and freedoms around what I can expect from the kitchen.

Once you know the list of foods from which she is abstaining, that food is out of the kitchen. You can have your own stash somewhere separate from her routine path. You can eat whatever you want, just not in front of her.

Quiz Question:

You live in the same house. You love ice cream, but she's abstinent from it. How can you still have ice cream?

Answer: You can store your ice cream at work. You can have ice cream on the way home from work. You can get a small freezer with a lock. Put it in your workshop or garage. Store and eat it there. Keep the freezer locked. Dispose of the container and clean up your bowls yourself. (Either put the container directly into the garbage can [hidden in a grocery sack], or take it with you when you leave the next day and toss it somewhere else.)

I truly want to help.

Then you are helping already by reading this book. The more you can embrace the idea that the goal is to decrease appetite chemicals and promote satiety chemicals, the more your behavior will be guided by wisdom and the strategies you've learned in this book. That is a huge gift.

I want to be eating healthier myself.

These principles can work for you too. If you just want to spruce up your food plan, eating small snacks, a bit of protein with every meal or snack, and staying away from neurotoxins will help you.

If you suspect you also have an appetite disorder or a food addiction, then you'll need the other book, *Your Appetite Switch*. I've put information and tips in that book that I haven't bothered you with here, because that degree of detail isn't necessary in order for you to support her. But if you have similar issues, then you'll need to know which of your own chemicals are out of balance, how to promote serotonin, and in which order to make changes.

I want to stay with my own eating plan when her eating gets wild.

It truly is a challenge to not get sucked into someone else's relapse, especially if she wants company in it. Here's what to do. Tell her, "Honey, I would like your support as I maintain my own eating program. I have a great book that will tell you how to support me. Will you read it?"

Then hand her this book.

I want relief from worrying about her health.

If she is not on a food plan or working with a recovery program, does she want to be? If so, then you can offer her *Your Appetite Switch* so that she will have a systematic way to turn off her appetite.

Perhaps, though, you've made lots of suggestions over the years and she has only resisted them. You have some options.

Option 1: Tell her that you understand now why diets have never worked for her in the past, and that your heart goes out to her for all the effort she's made, considering that diets can't be the solution for an overactive appetite. Assure her that you are interested only because you love her and want the best for her. Ask if she'd be willing to at least take a look at this book, to see why she hasn't failed, but that diets have failed her.

Option 2: The most effective tool, if a person is either highly resistant or deeply trapped by an addiction, is an intervention. An intervention is a tightly structured, planned meeting of concerned friends and family that can be led by a professional. There are professionals trained in the art of intervention, and their guidance can make all the difference.

I just googled the word intervention and found 64 million responses, so that's one place to start. Even though most on the list are concerned with alcohol or drug intervention, the principles are exactly the same with food addiction. Talk to a few practitioners and find one who can see the parallels.

A fine book on the subject is *Living on the Edge: A Guide to Intervention for Families With Drug and Alcohol Problems* by Katherine Ketcham and Ginny Lyford Gustafson.

I want to be able to share more experiences with her.

What is in the way? The eating, the addiction, or has she pulled away from you in order to protect herself from people who don't understand food addiction or appetite disorder?

Talk to her. Discuss what's in the way of sharing more experiences. Let her know what you've been learning. Find out if she wants your help. Decide how much help you want to offer.

Are there activities or jaunts you would like to share with her that get curtailed or cancelled because of her eating, weight, shame, or body image?

Shame

Sometimes a person is reluctant to enter the public arena out of shame over weight or a fear of being shamed. To discuss this with her requires tact and delicacy. Approach the issue from your desire to be with her. See if there are ways to reduce some of the restraining factors.

Shame is a slow death. It disables us as effectively as leg-irons. A protocol for undoing shame is in my book, *When Misery is Company*.

Fear of Being Shamed

Be willing to become a secret service agent against abuse. If someone makes a mean comment, defend her. If someone stares at her, stare back.

I'm fierce when I am in public with an obese friend. I often go first and if someone stares, I stare them down before she even notices.

I love what one friend said when a stranger demeaned his obese daughter. He said in very firm tones, "Are you speaking about *my* daughter?" And the bully mumbled an apology and backed away.

If someone is malicious, the worst response is to pretend it didn't happen. This tactic has the effect of isolating each of the good people in the situation. She's hurt, you and your friends are pretending, and a pall is now over the event as you try to have fun when each of you has a rock in your gut.

You already know how to handle a mean family member. If a stranger is cruel, turn to your friend and say, "I'm so sorry that creep said that. I am furious at his ignorance. What about you? Are you mad or hurt?" This allows everyone to experience the comfort of solidarity.

Unreadiness

My beloved friend was in a transition. After a lifetime of being able to go anywhere she wanted, obesity was beginning to put her on the sidelines. She wanted to go to a concert but the distance from the parking area to the concert hall was further than she could walk.

I was afire with solutions and finally she just got irritated with me. She couldn't go, she insisted. She shut me up with some pointed sentences.

She'd given up on the idea, and I had to accept it. Some time later she did get a wheelchair and we did go to a concert together. She wasn't ready until then, and my fervor could not make her ready.

Body Image Issues

People can imagine themselves the size of an elephant even if they're not overweight or only slightly larger than normal. (Although normal in the United States—with 65% of the population overweight—*is* to carry extra pounds.)

A person can be shackled by her image of herself regardless of the reality, and it can interfere with a willingness to try things. One of my friends once said that she wouldn't let herself kayak until she had lost weight. There was no reason for her to deny herself kayaking. Kayaks, like shirts, come in lots of sizes. There was no physical reason for her to not try it, but she was accustomed to withholding life from herself.

I've heard countless stories of women depriving themselves from life experience out of fear of not fitting—a wetsuit, a life jacket, a seat, a group, a club—or out of the fear of trying to fit while others are watching. (If this is the case, call the business in question and gather data—how wide are the seats, is there a weight limit, do you have a private room where she can try on the special clothing?)

Limited Sight Distance

The above issues have this in common: the person is deep inside her own view of herself, unable to comprehend a different perspective. For example, if she is convinced that everyone stares at her because of her weight, she may be unable to take in the reality that no one is paying her any attention. She has a perspective that causes her to distort the actual data.

One way to see if you can soften this boundary is to ask, "What are the losses for you if you hold tight to this viewpoint?" Then wait and use compassionate listening as she answers.

Then ask, "Can you open yourself to a difference in the way I see this?" And ask her to listen compassionately to you.

Choosing Food Over Life

Just as an alcoholic can miss a lot of life hanging out in a bar, a deeply entrenched food addiction can hold a person's focus to eating rather than living. Once you've followed any suggestions here that match your level of investment, you may have to let go of your hopes for the person you love.

If she's been shown wider options, it is, ultimately, her decision.

34

Give the Dragon Its Own Subgroup

The family drew near the old farmhouse in high spirits. We drove up as Aunt Gloria lugged a huge basket of exotic fare up the porch steps. I laughed as Papa Blaine called quips from the porch.

My mate and I looked at each other and I gave her a thumbs-up. I got her snacks and our cooler, and held her hand as we entered the dining room. The old oak table was groaning with bowls of potatoes and biscuits, jam and candied yams, sweet cranberry jelly and baskets of yeast rolls.

I grabbed mom and grandma and pulled them into a corner after giving each a big hug. I reminded them that she was in good recovery from her appetite disorder and deserved all our support. I asked permission to rearrange the table and to add our own specially cooked foods.

Mom was worried that the symmetry of the table would be destroyed, but Grandma came through with, "Symmetry, schmitry, let the boy take care of his wife."

Grandma helped me move all the sugary and starchy dishes to the other end of the table. We made a little sugar-free zone with a warmer that held our own baked yams, our wild rice dressing, and our own gravy. We put out a large bowl of natural-made cranberry sauce, enough for everyone to try.

I braved the kitchen and transferred our homemade whipping cream and ice cream to the fridge. Our containers bore stickers that warned, "Hands Off, Special Healthnut Food."

My sister, Barbara, had already agreed to sit on the other side of my wife so that she'd be fenced away from the immediate smell and sight of sugary and starchy foods. Barbara was experimenting with some of our same eating changes and was enthusiastic about helping.

Finally, all was ready and the whole crowd gathered at the large family table. Everyone took a seat and, one by one, each selection was passed around. We were at the end of the table with Grandma across from us. When contraband was passed to me, I just handed it across to Grandma who fielded it down the other side. This way, my wife never had to handle platters of addictive food.

We all dug in. Uncle Mean, already one sheet to the wind, called, "What's with you at the end of the table. Too good to associate with us?"

"Hey, Uncle Mean," I said, "Want another glass of wine? I brought a good Chablis."

"Sure, Guy, you always were my favorite nephew."

I handed him the bottle and, tension diverted, we continued our meal in comfortable chaos.

When dessert time arrived, Aunt Milli became an unexpected ally. She brought out two different cobblers, one of which was sugar and flour free. We fell over her with gratitude. "Aunt Milli, how come you went to this extra trouble?"

She smiled shyly, "I just wanted to support your wife and since Grandma was diagnosed with diabetes, I thought maybe we could all learn from what you are doing."

Cousin Snide brought the other desserts out from the kitchen and remarked, "I don't suppose you're going to have any of Great Grandma's pies, even though she wielded the rolling pin herself with her weak, arthritic fingers."

"You're so perceptive, Cousin Snide. We did bring our own pumpkin pie and though we're willing to share, we know Great Grandma's pies are the best, so don't feel that you're hurting our feelings if you choose to eat hers."

We cut wedges of our own sugar-free pie and dressed it with our own sugar-free toppings. Aunt Loving called, "Guy, cut me a sliver of your pie. If I can learn to eat as well as you two do, it would be good for me."

Joan and Blaine joined in, and so did Sherry, and soon we had a sugar-free pie-eating subgroup. The other pie eaters were content with their desserts and we were content with ours.

It was our best Thanksgiving yet.

❦ Thanksgiving Menu ❦

Appetizer
Cheese Cuke Sandwiches*

Salad
Mixed greens with Balsamic Vinegrette
or
Lettuce Wedges with Blue Cheese Sprinkles

Main Course
Natural Roast Turkey
Wild Rice Stuffing
Natural Cranberry Sauce
Mashed Potatoes or Potato Yam Swirl
Baked Yams
Green Beans with Bacon or Roasted Pepper Garnish
Calm White Gravy
Baked Vidalias*

Dessert
Anne's Famous Pumpkin Pie with spelt almond Crust
Oatmeal Cobbler*
Homemade Ice Cream*
Maple Whipped Cream

*Optional items

Appendix A
Recipes

Suggestions

Amend recipes to take into account your family's food allergies.

Adjust both recipes and your shopping list according to the flours, oils, and sweeteners she is now using.

Shopping—Some stores shelve healthy oils and whole grain flours with standard items, and others have a special section for healthy foods. If you can't find the recommended item among like products, look for it in the health food aisles.

Be sure that you pick ingredients and foods that have no msg, aspartame, equal, nutraSweet, or sugar. This includes canned green beans, chicken broth, turkey, dried cranberries.

Information
All recipes serve 8 people.

You can find a shopping list and other recipes at www.master**your**appetite.com.

* This item is optional

++This item can be prepared in advance.

Special Instructions

You must revise these recipes when the ingredients listed are your loved one's shotgun trigger foods. The goal is to have a lovely holiday dinner without disrupting her abstinence. You are seeking a balance between providing all the traditional favorites so that she doesn't feel deprived, while keeping the consciousness that this is just one day, and one day is not worth losing abstinence.

Stuffing and Rolls.

Two traditional items are glaringly omitted: bread stuffing and rolls. If she isn't abstinent from bread yet, then you can make traditional dressing, but use Ezekiel or sprouted wheat bread instead of ordinary bread. If she is abstinent from bread, then even these substitutions run the risk of destroying her abstinence.

Bread is very hard to give up and just one roll will break abstinence. Once broken, it can be months or years before she will regain bread abstinence. There is no substitution for rolls that won't trigger. Not sprouted wheat, Ezekiel rolls, potato rolls, whole wheat rolls, sour dough, or alternative flour rolls. It's better to simply not have any kind of roll, biscuit, or bread on her part of the table.

Flour and Thickeners

The only time wheat flour is used in any of the following recipes is for pie crust. If she is abstinent from all wheat, use the no-wheat pie crust recipe. If she's abstinent from all flour, use the flourless pie crust recipe. Or bake the pumpkin filling as you would a custard and serve it without any crust at all.

When recipes call for flour, use potato or brown rice flour for savory recipes and tapioca flour for sweet recipes. If she is abstinent from all flour, use cornstarch as a thickener. If she is abstinent from corn, use arrowroot or egg yolks. Arrowroot thickens at a lower temperature than flour and the gravy or sauce must be used immediately. It will not reheat.

Egg yolks should not be added directly to hot liquid but blended into evaporated milk first. Add some of the warm sauce to this mixture, and then add this mixture to the rest of the sauce which has been allowed to cool and is now over a low heat. Stir it in gradually. Do not let it boil. (A double boiler removes the suspense and doesn't punish you if you get distracted with something else.)

Sweeteners

Here you must tread carefully. If she is abstinent from sugar, but not from honey, and if items baked with honey do not trigger her, then you can use the recipes as is. However, if she is abstinent from honey, then substitute with maple syrup or fruit concentrate. You can make fruit concentrate by boiling apples, pears, or grapes to a thick syrup. If she is abstinent from these, then the cranberry sauce can be sweetened with stevia. Add drops of stevia to taste after all cooking is done and before refrigerating.

The pie depends on a sweetener for bulk and texture, not just for taste, so if she's abstinent from all syrups and concentrates, then you may have to resort to splenda. Never, under any circumstances, use equal or NutraSweet.

Substitutions:
Maple syrup
Fruit concentrate
Molasses
Splenda

Fat Abstinence

If she is abstinent from butter, substitute oil. Use sesame oil for sweet recipes and sesame, peanut, or olive oil for savory recipes. For the pie crust, use lard or shortening instead of butter.

Cheese Cuke Sandwiches

Cucumber
Havarti cheese, 1 package
*Dill
Seasoning
*Olives or roasted peppers, small jar
toothpicks

Wash cucumber. Peel the skin if it's bitter.
Slice thinly. Spread on paper towel. Chill.
Slice Havarti thinly. Place cheese slice between two cucumber slices. Sprinkle cheese lightly with dill or seasoning.
Skewer with toothpick on which a half olive or roasted pepper piece has been threaded.

Mixed Green Salad

Mixed Greens, 1 bag
Vinaigrette, 1 bottle
*Mushroom pieces, dried (unsweetened) cranberries, and/or soy nuts, 1/4 cup
*Roasted garlic, 2 T
*Sliced celery, 1 stalk
*Grated carrot, one
*Onion slivers, 2T

Wash bag of mixed greens thoroughly, rinsing and draining at least twice. (Prepared greens can have high bacteria counts. Even if they are pre-washed, they must be washed again before serving.)
Add any optional ingredients.
At the last minute, drizzle with vinaigrette.

++Vinaigrette

Olive and/or sesame oil, 3/4 cup
Balsamic Vinegar, 1/2 cup
Garlic, 2 smashed cloves, or 5 minced roasted garlic cloves
*Asiago or parmesan cheese, 1/4 cup
*Salt and pepper, to taste

Whisk or shake all ingredients together, or blend briefly at high speed. Store in a covered container.

Lettuce Wedges

Lettuce, 1 head
Lettuce Dressing
*Blue cheese pieces
*Toasted almonds

Wash lettuce. Chill.
Slice into sizable wedges. Place each wedge on a separate plate.
Drizzle each wedge with Lettuce Dressing, or mayonnaise thinned with buttermilk or milk.
*Dust with blue cheese sprinkles
*Dust with roasted almond pieces

++Lettuce Dressing

Mayonnaise, 3/4 cup
Ketchup, 1/2 cup
Mustard, 1/4 cup
*Horseradish, 1T

Mix ingredients until smooth.

Natural Roast Turkey

Safety pins
White 100% cotton fabric, 10 X 12 inches
Natural Turkey or turkey breast—if possible, one that has never been frozen.

(Be sure *not* to get any turkey that has been injected. Msg or other flavor enhancers and some form of sugar are a part of injected solutions, ruining an otherwise nearly perfect food. Natural turkeys do cost more, but compared to eating out, they are still a good value. They also taste considerably better.)

2-4 days ahead:

If the turkey is frozen, begin defrosting in refrigerator. (Fresh turkey that has never been frozen is noticeably tastier.)

Thanksgiving morning:

Remove the turkey from the refrigerator an hour or two in advance and let it come to room temperature. Wash inside and out and remove the giblets. (If your family likes giblets, cook them and add them to dressing or gravy. If not, boil and cut them up for the animals that can tolerate rich food.)

Preheat oven to 450°. While it's warming, pick out about 8 of the largest safety pins. Boil them in a pan of water.

++Cut a rectangle of white 100% cotton fabric and wash in hot sudsy water. Rinse it well in cold water. Let it air dry.

Stuff turkey with wild rice dressing. Close with safety pins. Rub turkey with shortening. Place turkey in oven and immediately reduce heat to 350°.

Soak the cotton rectangle in unsalted shortening. Place on turkey breast after the first hour of cooking.

Baste occasionally. Bake for recommended cooking time, adding 5 min. per pound if stuffed.

++*Wild Rice Stuffing*

Wild and/or brown basmati rice, 6 cups when cooked
Natural chicken broth, 2 quarts
Celery, chopped, 1 cup
Onion, chopped, 1/2 cup
*Garlic, minced, 1-2 cloves
*Apple, 1
*Raisins, 1/4 cup
*Pecans, 1/2 cup
*Mushrooms, sautéed, 1 cup
Seasonings
*Paprika, 1/4 t

Wash and drain wild or mixed wild and brown rice. Follow package directions to produce 6 cups of rice, substituting chicken broth for water. *Use organic or natural chicken broth that has no msg or sugar added, such as Pacific Natural Foods chicken broth.*

In a separate saucepan, heat 1 cup of broth. In it, cook until soft:

- celery
- onion
- garlic*

When rice is fully cooked, mix in celery and onion. You may also add any combination of the optional ingredients. Season.

If prepared ahead, warm mixture before stuffing bird.

++Natural Cranberry Sauce

Prepare at least one day before Thanksgiving.
Cranberries, 3 cups or 12 oz
Orange juice, 3/4 cup
Gelatin, 1 package
Honey, 1/4 cup
*Tangerine segments

Wash, pick off stems, and drain cranberries.
Boil with:

1/2 cup water
1/2 cup orange juice
1/4 cup honey (if it is a nontriggering sweetener)

When skins split, put mixture through a food mill unless you want whole berry sauce. Boil another ten minutes.

While boiling cranberries, soften 1 package of gelatin on 1/4 cup of orange juice. Turn off heat under cranberries when boiling is completed and add gelatin to mixture. Stir until gelatin is dissolved. Pour into 1.5 quart heat tolerant bowl and refrigerate when cool.

If using splenda, add it with the softened gelatin.

*Garnish with tangerine segments in a sunburst design.

Mashed Potatoes

Potatoes, 6-8 white or Yukon gold
Cream cheese or Neufchatel, 1/2 pound
Butter
Salt, 1t or to taste
*Garlic powder, 1t
*Paprika
*Parsley

Peel and chop white potatoes into large wedges. Boil until soft in lightly salted water. Drain.

Meanwhile, in large bowl, put:

> Neufchatel or cream cheese
> Salt
> Garlic powder*
> 1 tsp paprika*

Add potatoes to bowl and mash, whip, or blend. Garnish with pats of butter and/or parsley.

Potato Yam Swirl

Yams or sweet potatoes, 4
Neufchatel or cream cheese, 1/4 pound
Salt, 1/2 t

Halve mashed potato recipe. Peel and chop yams or sweet potatoes and boil until soft. Drain. Mash, whip, or blend with 1/4 pound cream or Neufchatel cheese and 1/2 tsp salt. Stir into mashed potatoes with a swirling pattern.

Baked Yams

Yams or sweet potatoes
Cinnamon
Nutmeg

Wash yams or sweet potatoes well. Scrape off unsavory spots. Bake in 400° oven for 1 hour. After 30 minutes, pierce each potato a couple of times with a fork. When baked, cut into the top lengthwise and squeeze from the ends. Sprinkle lightly with cinnamon or very lightly with nutmeg.

Green Beans

Green Beans, 1 large can or 1 pound of fresh beans
Broth
Vinegar, 1T
*Roasted red pepper bits or bacon crumbles

Open and drain can of green beans. If sugar has been added, rinse and drain again. Or wash and snap raw beans.

Heat in broth till just tender. Sprinkle with vinegar. *Garnish with chopped roasted red pepper or bacon crumbles.

Calm White Gravy

Potato flour
Neufchatel or cream cheese, 1/2 pound
Evaporated milk, 1 can
Salt and pepper
Remove a cup of turkey drippings from roasting pan while turkey is cooking. Chill and remove the fat from the top. In a skillet or saucepan, warm 4 tablespoons of potato flour at low heat. Add about 4 tablespoons of the defatted drippings and whip until flour is blended. Do not allow the flour to cook or fry. As soon as the flour is creamy, add 1/2 pound of Neufchatel or cream cheese and the rest of the defatted drippings. Blend and heat. As the flour thickens, add evaporated milk gradually, until you have about 2 cups of gravy at the desired consistency. Salt and pepper to taste.

*Baked Vidalia's

Sweet onions, 8
Butter or oil
Parmesan-shredded, 4 oz
*Salt and pepper

Pre-heat oven to 375°. Peel sweet onions, preferably Vidalia's or Walla Walla's.

(Vidalia season is long gone by November, so I buy a bag of Vidalia's at the end of the growing season, and spread them out over wire mesh in the coolest, darkest part of the basement. Some will begin to rot, but if all rot is cut off, the rest of the onion can be salvaged. Do not store onions and potatoes near each other.)

Place in a baking dish and dot with butter or sprinkle olive or sesame oil over each onion. Salt very lightly. Grind pepper over top if desired.

Bake an hour and a half. The moment you remove them from the oven, sprinkle with shredded parmesan.

Anne's Famous Pumpkin Pie

Pumpkin, either 15 oz can or ++*3 cups from baked fresh pumpkin
Honey, 1/2 cup
Molasses, 1/4 cup
Evaporated milk, 1 can
Salt, 1t
Cinnamon, 2t
Ginger, 1t
Clove, 1/2t
Vanilla, 1t
2 eggs, beaten (canned pumpkin), 5 eggs, beaten (fresh pumpkin)
*Pecans, whole, 1/2 cup
Pie crust

Makes1- 2 pies. Preheat oven 425°. Check warning about sweeteners and substitute as needed.

[*++Fresh pumpkin: Halve or quarter a medium-size pumpkin. Scoop out seeds and strings. (You can set seeds aside and bake on a cookie sheet for a healthy snack.) Bake pumpkin meat at 375° until tender, 1-1.5 hours. Scrape meat away from skin.]

Combine all ingredients above the line. Place pecans on the piecrust before filling with pumpkin mixture. After filling, garnish with pecans in an interesting pattern. Bake at 425° for 15 minutes, then 350° for 40-50 minutes. (Fresh pumpkin takes longer, sometimes as much as 20-30 minutes, so check every 10 minutes.) Remove when an inserted knife comes out clean.

++Spelt Almond Pie Crust
Mix:
> 1 1/2 cups spelt flour
> 1/4 cup sorghum flour
> 1 cup brown rice flour
> 1/4 cup almonds crushed fine but not paste
> 1 tsp gran marcilla (Has strong flavor. Be sure you
like it.)
> or 1 tsp cinnamon

Work into mixture:
> 2/3 cup cold butter

Chill. Mix in:
> 6-8 T ice cold water

And roll out, then shape into pie pan. Chill, then fill with pumpkin mixture. Arrange whole pecans in a circle on top.

Whipping Cream
Whipping cream
Maple syrup or stevia
Vanilla, 1t

> In a large tall-sided bowl, pour whipping cream. Whip with a blender until stiff. Add 2 T of maple syrup or a couple of drops of stevia and 1 tsp vanilla. Blend about 10 seconds.

*Oatmeal Cobbler
Apples and/or peaches or pears, 3-4 cups,
Honey
Tapioca, 2T
Cinnamon
Salt
Vanilla, 1t
Potato or tapioca flour
Honey or maple syrup
Maple syrup or molasses
Oatmeal, 1 cup
Baking powder
Butter, melted, 1/2 cup
Pam

Preheat oven 350°.

Wash, core, and slice fruit. Mix with:

> 1/2 cup honey
> 2 T tapioca

Let stand, covered for at least 15 minutes. Add:

> 1 tsp cinnamon
> 1/8 tsp salt
> 1 tsp vanilla
> 2 T potato flour
> 2 T honey or maple syrup

Spread across a baking dish coated with Pam. Heat till boiling hot.

Mix:

> 1 cup oatmeal
> 1/2 cup spelt, potato, or tapioca flour
> 1/2 cup honey
> 1/4 cup maple syrup or molasses
> 1/4 tsp salt
> 1/4 tsp baking powder

Add 1/2 cup butter. Mix and sprinkle across the top of the hot fruit.

Bake 30-35 minutes, till brown.

++ *Ice Cream

For this you will need an ice cream maker. For small makers, make two batches to serve 8. Store in the freezer in ice cube trays. Do not leave it in one bowl. It will freeze too hard to be scooped. The ice cube trays let you pop them out in serving sizes for pie or cobbler a la mode.

Blend and chill:

> 3 cups half and half or milk
> 4 oz egg beaters
> 2 T maple syrup
> 1 T vanilla

Pour into ice cream maker and follow maker instructions.

Leftovers

One the best things about Thanksgiving is leftovers, but if your food addict is abstinent from bread, will she miss out on those wonderful turkey sandwiches?

Not entirely. Depending on her degree of abstinence, she may still be able to have wraps or pocket bread without getting triggered. These wraps should be low carb, wheat free, or whole wheat, depending on where she's set her boundary.

For a complete shopping list and additional recipes, go to www.masteryourappetite.com.

Appendix B
Resources

O-Anon

PO Box 1314
North Fork, CA 93643 USA
Phone: (559) 877-3615
Email: oanon@netptc.net

Support for the family and friends of overeaters.

Al-Anon

Al-Anon Family Group Headquarters, Inc.
1600 Corporate Landing Parkway
Virginia Beach, VA 23454-5617
Phone: (757) 563-1600
Email: wso@al-anon.org
http://www.al-anon.alateen.org

Support for the family and friends of alcoholics.

SCT®

Systems-Centered Training
www.systemscentered.com
admin@systemscentered.com

Training for helping professionals and organizational consultants in the art of human system development with workshops and training that are open to the public.

SSA/MAA
Self Sabotagers Anonymous
(Formerly Misery Addicts Anonymous)
Email: info@miseryaddicts.org
www.miseryaddicts.org

A 12-step program for those who sabotage themselves or who fear success.

Anne Katherine
www.master**your**appetite.com

Telephone and online programs for people with a malfunctioning appetite switch.

Appendix C
Notes

Chapter 4

[i] SP Kalra, PS Kalra, "Neuropeptide Y: a physiological orexigen modulated by the feedback action of ghrelin and leptin." *Endocrine*, Oct;22(1)2003m 49-56

[ii] G Williams, JA Harrold, and DJ Cutler, "The hypothalamus and the regulation of energy homeostasis: lifting the lid on a black box." *Proceedings of the Nutrition Society*, Aug;59(3)2000:385-96.

[iii] NPY, ghrelin, Orexins A & B, Dopamine, Norepinephrine, dynorphin, endorphins

Chapter 7

[iv] RL Batterham & SR Bloom, "The gut hormone peptide YY regulates appetite." *Annals of the New York Academy of Sciences.* 2003 Jun;994:162-8.

[v] IBID

[vi] CJ Small & SR Bloom, "Gut hormones and the control of appetite." *Trends in Endocrinology and Metabolism.* 2004 Aug;15(6):259-63.

[vii] RL Batterham, M. A. Cohen, S. M. Ellis, C. W. Le Roux, D. J. Withers, G. S. Frost, M. A. Ghatei, et al, "Inhibition of food intake in obese subjects by peptide YY_{3-36}," *New England Journal of Medicine*, 2003 Sept;349(10):941-948

[viii] SJ Konturek, J. W. Konturek, T. Pawlik, T. Brzozowski, et al. "Brain-gut axis and its role in the control of food intake." *Journal of Physiology and Pharmacology* 2004, 55(1)"137-154

Chapter 9

[ix] Nora D. Volkow, Gene-Jack Wang, Joanna S. Fowler, Jean Logan, Millard Jayne, Dinko Franceschi, Cristopher Wong, Samuel J. Gatley, Andrew N. Gifford, Yu-Shin Ding, Naomi Pappas, "Nonhedonic food motivation in humans involves dopamine in the dorsal striatum and methylphenidate amplifies this effect," *Synapse,* 2002 June; Vol. 44, Issue 3.

Chapter 12

[x] Schematic of Hypothalamus from Hanaway, Joseph, et al, *Brain Atlas*, Fitzgerald Science Press, Bethesda, 1998, page 231. Permission granted by John Wiley & Sons, Inc. Global Rights Dept., 2008.

Chapter 13

[xi] Some research shows low circulating blood levels of leptin with anorexia and bulimia and high levels with binge eating, but these studies did not check for receptor sensitivity. If leptin is high, but receptors aren't taking any messages, it could explain these contradictory results.

[xii] Konturek, as cited in Chapter 11, p149.

[xiii] J. Sanchez, P. Oliver, A. Palou, C. Pico. "The inhibition of gastric ghrelin production by food intake in rats is dependent on the type of macronutrient," *Endocrinology*, 2004, Nov;145(11): 5049-55.

[xiv] Konturek, as cited in Chapter 11.

Chapter 15

[xv] Russell Blaylock, *Excitotoxins, the Taste that Kills*, Health Press, NM, 1997.

[xvi] All of the content on this and the next page has been derived from *Excitotoxins* by Russell Blaylock.

[xvii] Olney, JW. "Brain lesions, obesity, and other disturbances in mice treated with monosodium glutamate." *Science*, 1969 May;164(880):719-21

[xviii] Blaylock, *Excitotoxins*, see footnote 2 or http://www.healthpress.com

[xix] Dawson, R, et al. "Attenuation of leptin-mediated effects by monosodium glutamate-induced arcuate nucleus damage." *American Journal of Physiology*. 1997 jul;273(1 Pt 1):E202-6

Chapter 18

[xx] 1999-2000 National Health and Nutrition Examination Survey, National Center for Health Statistics, CDC, www.cdc.gov

[xxi] p. 131, C. Davis, S. Strachan, and M. Berkson, "Sensitivity to reward: implications for overeating and overweight." *Appetite.* 2004, Apr;42(2):131-8

[xxii] G. J. Wang, N. D. Volkow, P. K. Thanos, and J. S. Fowler, "Similarity between obesity and drug addiction as asessed by neurofunctional imaging; a concept review," *Journal of Addictive Diseases.* 2004;23(3)'39-53

[xxiii] C. M. Cannon and M. R. Bseikri, "Is dopamine required for natural reward?" *Physiology and Behavior.* 2004 Jul;81(5):741-8.

[xxiv] G. Meyer, J. Schwertfeger, M. S. Exton, O. E. Janssen, W. Knapp, M.A, Stadler, M. Schedlowski, T.H. Kruger, "Neuroendocrine response to casino gambling in problem gamblers," *Psychoneuroendocrinology.* 2004 Nov;29(10):1272-80.

[xxv] Anne Katherine, *How to Make Almost Any Diet Work* , Hazelden, MN, 2006, pp 5-6

Chapter 25

[xxvi] Anthony Cincotta, Shugin Luo, Ying Zhang, Yin Liang, Keshavan bina Thomas Jetton, Piotr Seislowski, Chronic infusion of norepinephrine into the VMH of normal rats induces the obese state, *American Journal of Physiology—Regulatory, Integrative and Comp Physiology,* 2000 Feb; 278(2), 435-444.

[xxvii] Ibid

[xxviii] Ibid

[xxix] Ibid

[xxx] Ibid

[xxxi] Ibid

[xxxii] Kelli Taylor, Erin Lester, Bryan Hudson, Sue Ritter, Hypothalamic and hindbrain NPY, AGRP and NE increase consummatory feeding responses. *Physiology and Behavior.* 2007 Jan 4; : 17289093 (P,S,E,B,D)

[xxxiii] Amy Amsten, Rex Matthew, Ravi Ubriani, Jane Taylor, Bao-Ming Li, "Alpha-1 noradrenergic receptor stimulation impairs prefrontal cortical cognitive function," *Biological Psychiatry,* 1999, Jan; 45(1): 26-31.

xxxiv This term comes from Systems-Centered® Training. SCT® and Systems-Centered® are registered trademarks of Dr. Yvonne M. Agazarian and the Systems-Centered Training and Research Institute, Inc., a non-profit organization.

Chapter 27

xxxv A brief history: Therapeutic listening has been around as a purposeful therapeutic tool since the mid-twentieth century, when process-centered learning was advanced by Alfred North Whitehead, Carl Rogers, and a series of studies at the University of Chicago having to do with efficacy of therapeutic methods. Eventually this work changed the face of psychotherapy and spread among practitioners in many helping disciplines.

xxxvi The works of Laura Rice, Eugene Gendlin, Marge Felder, and Marshall Rosenberg were fruits of these studies. Their books still offer valuable information.

xxxvii Functional subgrouping is part of an entire system of defense modification developed by Dr. Yvonne Agazarian, equally brilliant as both theorist and therapist.

xxxviii SCT® and Systems-Centered® are registered trademarks of Dr. Yvonne M. Agazarian and the Systems-Centered Training and Research Institute, Inc., a non-profit organization.

xxxix Fortunately, therapists in Canada, the United States, England, and Scandanavia are being trained by her firsthand, so you may be able to find a Systems-Centered practitioner near you, should you be interested in expanding what I offer here.

xl Agazarian, Y.M. (1997). Systems-centered therapy for groups. New York: Guilford Press. Re-printed in paperback (2004). London: Karnac Books.

xli The entire process described here comes from Systems-Centered® Training, developed by Dr. Yvonne Agazarian and SCTRI. SCT® and Systems-Centered® are registered trademarks of Dr. Yvonne M. Agazarianand the Systems-Centered Training and Research Institute, Inc., a non-profit organization. For more information, see www.systemscentered.com

Appendix D
Index

Appendix E
Meet Anne Katherine

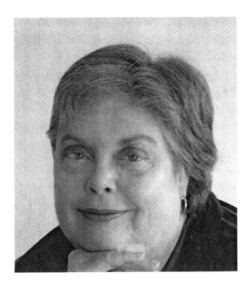

Anne Katherine—best-selling author, respected therapist, and a recovering overeater.   From a radio interview, Anne's words, "Food ran my life until I found recovery, and then I wanted answers. I was convinced that something had driven my eating.

"It couldn't have been my conscious choice to be preoccupied with food when I was five or ten years old. Something in my body was responding to something in food."

This passion for solutions led her to 30 years of research and a specialty in treating overeating in her practice north of Seattle. Now she trains therapists, leads retreats and workshops, and conducts her streamlined program, Master Your Appetite, that is available for people anywhere in the world.

Anne Katherine is a Certified Eating Disorders Specialist, an MA psychologist, and a Board certified regression therapist. She has been practicing in hospital, agency, and private professional settings for 34 years.

Her attunement to her client's issues has again and again pushed her to the front line of psychological discovery where she has pioneered solutions for problems not yet articulated by anyone else. She wrote the first complete book on boundaries and wrote about food addiction, its chemical causes, and how to treat it long before most professionals were even recognizing it as a condition. She was the first to identify misery addiction and a process to recover from compulsive self-sabotage, and identified appetite disorder as the actual cause of most overeating.

Her books include *Boundaries, Anatomy of a Food Addiction, Where to Draw the Line, When Misery is Company, Penumbra: a Soul's Journey,* and *How to Make Almost Any Diet Work.* Her companion book to this one, *Your Appetite Switch,* will be available soon. You can find her at www.annekatherine.org and her program at www.masteryourappetite.com.

Printed in the United States
219799BV00004B/14/P

9 781598 587135